Borderline Personality Disorder

The Ultimate guide to Overcome Depression, Post-Traumatic Stress, Bipolar, and Anxiety Disorders

I0416872

By Karen Shepard

Table of Contents

Introduction 6

Chapter 1: What is Borderline Personality Disorder 13

    Signs and Symptoms: A Summary.........................19

    Treatment Options: A Summary 29

    How Others Can Help...38

Chapter 2: Causes of Borderline Personality Disorder
....43

    Genetics 47

    Brain Abnormalities...50

    Neurobiological Factors 57

    Developmental Factors..62

    Other Factors 65

Chapter 3: Signs and Symptoms of Recognizing
Borderline Personality Disorder 72

    Emotional Symptoms 78

    Behavior Symptoms...84

    Self-harm...86

    Interpersonal Relationships 89

    Sense of Self 92

    Cognitions..95

Chapter 4: Diagnosis of the Disorder 103

    International Classifications................................107

Impulsive Type 108

Borderline Type 111

Millon's Subtypes 116

The Conclusion 119

Family Members... 121

Adolescence... 124

Diagnosing with Other Disorders 126

Mood disorders.. 130

Premenstrual Dysphoric Disorder 134

Axis II Disorders.. 136

Chapter 5: Management and Prognosis.................. 138

Management 139

Psychotherapy....................................... 140

Medications.. 150

Services 154

Prognosis 156

Epidemiology 163

Chapter 6: Steps to Take in Order to Deal with
Borderline Personality Disorder 167

What the Family Can Do 168

What the Person with Borderline Personality Can
Do 184

Chapter 7: Controversies with Borderline Personality
Disorder.. 205

Credibility in Terms of Testimony from Those with
Borderline Personality Disorder 206

Dissociation 207

Lying as a feature 211

Gender 216

Manipulative Behavior 223

Stigma 227

Physical Violence 229

Mental Healthcare Professionals 232

Terminology 235

Chapter 8: Society and Culture: How they have
portrayed this Disorder to the Mass Population 237

Television and Film 238

Literature 241

Conclusion 246

Introduction

The thoughts that surround personality disorders has gained a lot of stigma in recent years. Many people are scared by what they will have seen on television or in books and they will often see the person with the disorder not as someone they should associate with, but as someone who is to be feared because they are off or going to do something that is crazy. This guidebook is going to take a look into one of these personality disorders, borderline personality disorder, and help you to discover what it is, if you or a loved one has it, and that it is not the person who is strange and wrong, but the disorder that is preventing that person from living the life that they would like.

Chapter 1 starts out with a good summary on what this kind of personality disorder is about. It will take some time to look at a brief description of the signs and symptoms, some of the available treatment options, and even how others will be able to help. While there will be more discussed in other chapters about these things, this is a good summary to help you get started on the right foot with getting an understanding.

Chapter 2 then gets into the meat of the issue a bit more and talks about some of the causes that can start borderline personality disorder. This chapter talks about how it is not completely understood what causes this kind of disorder and how some facts can be present in those who do not have the disorder. Some of the factors that might be present in those with this disorder, especially if they are mixed together include genetics, brain abnormalities, neurobiological factors, developmental factors, as well as some other things.

One of the best ways that you are going to be able to determine if you or someone else has this kind of disorder is to look for some of the signs and symptoms. There are a lot of different symptoms that can be found with this disorder and this chapter is going to split them up into different categories to make it easier to see where each of them lie. Some of the different signs and symptoms that you will be able to see in a person who has this kind of disorder include emotional symptoms, behavior symptoms, self-harm, interpersonal relationship issues, issues with their own sense of self, and cognition problems.

Chapter 4 talks a bit about how this kind of disorder is going to be diagnosed and some of the ways that you will be able to get a diagnosis from the therapist. Some of the topics that will be discussed in this chapter include the subtypes of the disorder, when the disorder will show up, how to diagnose it when other disorders are present, and so on. One of the best things that a person with this disorder is going to be able to do for themselves is to get a diagnosis so that they can get the kind of treatment that they need. Unfortunately, this kind of help is not always available to patients because they are not diagnosed or they are not willing to get the help that is needed.

Chapter 5 talks about what is going to happen once a diagnosis is made and the client has agreed to get the help that they need. This chapter talks about the management and prognosis that will occur during this phase. For the most part, therapy is the best option and this is what is going to be recommended for most patients. There are some cases where the person is going to need some medications to help out though. These are not going to be used in place of the therapy thought; they are often used to treat a few of the symptoms of the disorder or to help out if there are some other issues that are at play and can make the treatment much more effective.

Next is chapter 6 and it is going to talk a bit about the steps that are going to need to be taken in order to properly deal with this kind of personality disorder. It is going to start out with some of the steps that the family will be able to do in order to help out their loved one with their personality disorder in order to help out with the treatment. It will then go into some more details about what a person who has the disorder is able to do in order to give themselves the best chance at recovery. Recovery is possible for those who have this disorder, but they need to be willing to work for it and keep working and trusting the therapist to see the best results.

Finally, chapter 7 is going to take a look at some of the controversies that come with this kind of disorder. There are many people who think that those with this disorder are big liars and that they either do not have the disorder or if they do, they are just going to lie about it to the therapist and will never be able to get healed the way that they should. This chapter will go on to talk about some of the stigma that can come with borderline personality disorder, and how society and culture has been portrayed to the mass population.

As you can see, there is a lot of information about this kind of disorder and it can be confusing. It does not help matters that some of the symptoms of this disorder are going to be similar to some of the other disorders that are out there so it is hard to recognize and diagnose the disorder in some people. Use this guidebook to start getting a better understanding of the disorder and to help those who may be going through the issue right now in their lives and simply need the right treatment and support in order to make things better.

Chapter 1: What is Borderline Personality Disorder

There are a lot of different disorders that a person is able to get in their lifetime. Some may have issues with wanting to have everything be in the proper place while others may not get along with others and so much more. But this book is not going to spend time talking and worrying about those kinds of disorders. Instead, it is going to spend a lot of time going on about the disorder that is known as borderline personality disorder.

Borderline personality disorder is actually a cluster B personality disorder and will be marked with impulsivity, instability, and the person is going to have troubles with their own self-image and interpersonal relationships. Basically, it is a mental illness that is going to cause some intense behaviors in the person who is suffering from them. The people who are undergoing this kind of disorder will find that they have severe problems determining what their self-worth is, engage in impulsive behaviors in the hopes of getting an adrenaline rush and without care to how much it could hurt them and others, and very intense mood swings for no reason. If you know someone who has this disorder, you will notice that all of their relationships are troubled, whether it is with parents, siblings, friends, love interests, or coworkers.

In most of the cases, the signs for this kind of disorder are going to appear during their childhood, but the issues are not going to be present until they get a little bit older and enter early adulthood. The treatments for this kind of condition are going to be hard and it is not going to be something that will be done in just a few days or even weeks; this condition is going to take many years to heal and many times it never happens.

So you may be curious as to what is causing this disorder to occur. Unfortunately, experts are not in agreement at the exact causes of borderline personality disorders. Some believe that there are some issues with the chemicals inside the brain, the ones that control your mood, and that these are to blame for some people developing the disorder. It also looks like this disorder is carried through families so if you have someone in your family tree that had the disorder, your risk of developing it may go up.

Often, you will find that this kind of personality disorder is going to appear when the person had a childhood trauma of some kind. This could include a death of a close relative or their parent, being neglected, or being severely abused. The risk becomes higher when the child who is going through this trauma also has issues with coping with the stresses and anxieties that are around them. What this means is that just because a child has had a trauma in their life during childhood does not mean that this trauma is going to make them have borderline personality disorder. It does increase the chances of that occurring, but basically if they have a lot of trouble with fears, dealing with things that are happening around them, and do not like change, it is more likely that they are going to develop the disorder if some trauma does occur in their childhood.

For the most part, those with this kind of disorder are not going to get the help that they need. They are not going to recognize that they have any issues at all and so they are not going to get any help. Also, they have pushed away a lot of their own loved ones to the point that they do not have a lot of people who are going to want to have anything to do with them. This makes it very unlikely that they are going to have someone see that there is a problem and will get them the help that they need. This means that the person with the disorder is probably going to go without treatment unless something else comes up and then they are going to be stuck with this condition for the rest of their lives.

For those who are lucky enough to get treatment, they need to be able and willing to take the treatment that they are given. Many of those with this condition are not able to trust their therapists or do not think that they are going to need to stick around for a long time in order to get it done and so they will not get the proper help and will fail. They are going to need to find a therapist who is willing to stick with them and help out and they will need a lot of support in order to get through this time and seek the help that they need. If they are able to do this, they are more than likely going to succeed since this is what the statistics have pointed out in the past for other patients.

The symptoms are important to look for so that those around the person can get them the help that they need. Most of the time, the sufferer is not going to be able to see that they have a problem and at times they may not admit that anything is wrong at all.

Signs and Symptoms: A Summary

Sometimes, the issues with this disorder are hard to discover because everyone has times when they are struggling with their behaviors and emotions at some point. The difference between those with this personality disorder and normal people is that normal people will get over the emotions within a few days or so. On the other hand, those with this disorder will have really severe forms of the problem and they will repeat over and over during a long period of time rather than just showing up and then going away shortly after. These symptoms are also going to be disrupting the lives of those with the disorder because they are so severe and occur so often.

There are a lot of issues that can arise when you are dealing with this kind of personality disorder. The issue that a lot of people have, which will be discussed a bit later in a following chapter, is that a lot of these symptoms will match up with other issues and other personality disorders. This can make it difficult sometimes to diagnose who has this kind of personality disorder and who might have another issue that is unknown. Some of the issues that you should watch out for when you are worried that someone is suffering from this kind of personality disorder include:

- Intense mood swings and emotions. These can show up in several ways. First the person may have something that they can be upset about, but the amount that they react to it is way out of line for what should be called for.

They will do this all of the time instead of just once and it really can't be explained away with they are having a bad day. Other times, there may be absolutely no cause for the intense mood swings and the person will just be extremely happy one minute, angry the next, sad the next, and so on.

- Impulsive and harmful behaviors—the person with this kind of personality disorder is going to enjoy going out and seeking some thrills, no matter how dangerous these tasks may be to them or to someone else. They might go out and perform reckless driving, have risky sex, spend a lot of money that they do not have all of the time, binge eat, and abuse various forms of substance abuse. These people are not thinking about the consequences that might occur with their actions and are only worried about the moment that they are having right then.

- Issues with their relationship—most of the people with personality disorders like this one are going to have issues with their personal relationships. It really does not matter with what part of their lives and they may not have close friends or family either. This is often due to the fact that the person with this kind of personality disorder is only going to see things as good or bad and they will not see things differently or that others have opinions that are valid and different from their own. Also, the opinion that they have of someone else is going to dramatically change over any little thing. At one minute they may think you guys are best friends, but the next you may have to back out of a date or a meeting because of your kids at home, and the person

22

with the personality disorder will start to see you as bad and want nothing to do with you. This makes it almost impossible for them to have relationships with anyone.

- Low self-worth—the reason for this is not fully understood but it could be because they have no one whom they can be close to or because the chemicals in the brain that are responsible for this part of their lives are not working properly. These people are going to feel a lot of the time that they are not worth anyone paying attention to them and they might wonder why anyone would want to be their friend. This can make it difficult to talk to them because they are not going to see the point and may not have a lot to say.

- A fear that is almost frantic of being abandoned or left alone—since this person is dealing with a low self-worth and does not have many relationships that are working well for them, they may fear that the few friends whom they do have are not going to be there when they need them. The person with this disorder may start to do things that are considered frantic in order to hold onto the ones who may be close to them. On the other end of the spectrum, they may also reject and push away others because they feel it is better to do this before the ones they love can do it to them.

- Aggressive behavior—remember with this that the person with the disorder is going through some intense moments at the time and they are not sure of who they can trust of what they should be doing. These mixed up emotions are going to cause them to act out in ways that are not common for the general populace. Many people with borderline personality disorder are going to exhibit this kind of aggressive behavior.

- Feeling alone and empty inside—this can be two fold. First, the person is going to feel this way because their emotions are all over and they do not feel like they are worth anything. The few people who are around them may make the person feel like they are not worthy of love so they will push them away. In addition, since the person is not able to hold onto relationships all that well, they may have some issues with feeling alone because they have no one who is there to help them out.

- Problems with violence and anger—in some cases you may think that you are dealing with a little child who has never been told the word no. This is because the person with the personality disorder is prone to getting very angry and since they do not know how to control or express the anger, it is going to

erupt in some temper tantrums that can be

violent. It is not that they are trying to act like

a little child, it is more that they are not sure

how to act in society and much like a little

child, they just explode with emotions that

they do not understand and do not know what

to do with.

- Hurting themselves—often those with

  borderline personality disorder will resort to

  causing themselves physical harm. This would

  include things such as burning or cutting

  themselves. This is going to be a repeat issues,

  but it may be hard to see because the person

  is going to be working to hide up the scars so

  that no one else is able to see what is going

  on. For example, they may wear long dress

  shirts, long pants, and refuse to be anywhere

that a lot of skin would be showing, such as a swimming pool.

- Suicide attempts as well as suicidal thoughts—this is not uncommon in someone with borderline personality disorder. These thoughts stem from their risky behavior, trouble with emotions, and the fact that they feel all alone in this world.

- Paranoia and losing touch with reality—the human mind is a social creature. It likes to be around others that it can have conversations with, laugh with, and have a good time. Doing this is kind of hard for the person with this kind of disorder. They are always feeling like they are alone and often they are the ones who destroy the relationships that they are in. This leaves them with very few options when it comes to being social with others. As a result, their brains may turn a bit against them, over time, and they may begin to feel like others are after them or that they are not quite in touch with their reality like they should be.

As you can see, a lot of these symptoms are the same ones that you will be able to find in other personality disorders. This is what makes it really difficult to figure out if you have this kind of disorder and which kind you may have if not. It is never a good idea to diagnose yourself or someone else with this kind of personality disorder because you could be wrong and then the wrong treatments are given. It is much better to visit a doctor if there is a possibility of this disorder being present so that the person with it can get the help that they need quickly.

Treatment Options: A Summary

Don't think that if you or someone you know has this disorder that there is not a way that they can be helped. There is a lot that can be done to help someone with this kind of personality disorder, but it is going to take some time and it is not something that is easy to do. In fact, even after the treatment has been given and considered successful, there is a high chance that the same symptoms to come back.

The main issue here is that the people with this kind of disorder have a lot of trouble forming the right kinds of relationships with the doctors and counselors who are trying to help them. They may be wary of these professionals or think that they are after something and so they will close up and not get the help that they will need. This does not mean that therapies cannot be tried and hoped for, but it is going to be difficult to get through the process.

Some of the different ways that you can work in order to control the issues with the disorder will take a lot of time. The treatment is most likely going to be for the long term and if it happens to be successful, it may be able to help with managing emotions, preventing harmful behaviors, and even reducing some of the symptoms. A few methods of treatment that are often used include:

- Therapy and counseling—it is critical that you find someone who is a professional in different personalities to help out with this. If you are the one who is suffering from the personality disorder, you need to find a person you can trust and build up a relationship with them. If someone else has the problem, see if you can find a professional that they can connect with on a personal level at least somewhat. This is sometimes a difficult thing to do because people with this kind of personality disorder are going to flip flop around with who they trust and like; one moment they may see that their counselor is a caring and helpful person and the next they think the person is cruel. But developing this strong bond is critical if you want to have any chance of a recovery.

- Medicines—in some cases, medicines will be attempting to help out with the various emotions that the person is going through. Some common medicines that may work, depending on the person, will include antipsychotics, mood stabilizers and antidepressants. These should be given along with the therapy and counseling talked about above. Both of these can work together to assist the person with the personality disorder learn how to properly treat and manage it.

- Healthy habits—it is a good idea to start implementing good and healthy habits into the life of the personal with this disorder. This would include things such as avoiding drugs and alcohol, getting plenty of sleep, exercising on a regular basis, and eating foods that are healthy. Why is this so important? Because when you live a healthy lifestyle, a lot of the anxiety and stress the person may have been feeling before is going to go away and this will help to make their symptoms less frequent as well as less severe.

Often the treatment that is given is going to those who are looking for it is therapy. This is the best option because it is not just going to mask up the way that the person is feeling, but it is going to allow them to talk through the issue, come to the realization that they have an issue, and then they will be able to take the action to make the situation better. It is never recommended that there is some treatment without the majority of it coming from therapy.

If medication is used, it is often used in conjunction with the therapy. It is a good option to use in order to cut out some of the other issues that might be present along with the personality disorder, such as depression, anxiety, or another kind of personality disorder. But this means that it should be used in order to help the therapy but it is not going to work if it is being used as the sole method of taking care of the condition and it should never be used in this way.

With the right frame of mind and help from some of these treatments, many of those with borderline personality disorder will be able to find some relief from the more harmful symptoms in about a year of beginning the treatment. This does not mean that everything is gone, but the person may be able to socialize with others and have relationships and they are less likely to try and hurt themselves. In addition about half of the people who went through treatment are able to be done with most of the bad behaviors with around 10 years of the treatment.

Most of the people who have gone through some form of treatment were able to get the help that they needed and they did not have any worries about relapsing. Of course, there are a few cases where this kind of relapse is going to happen, but it is not going to be as much as with those who never got any treatment. If the person is able to get on a treatment and stick with it, you will find that it is much easier to stay with the new life and not have to worry about the issues of this disorder.

But those who never get treatment are never going to be able to see the great results that you would like. They are not going to be able to treat it on their own at all and so their failure rate is guaranteed. On the other hand, the majority of those who are able to get the treatment and will stick with it will be able to get recovered over the right period of time and the longer they stick with it, the more likely it is that they are going to be able to get the recovery and better life that they need.

This shows that treatment can be an effective way to deal with this disorder, but it is important to notice that it is going to take a lot of work. While most people are able to get rid of the symptoms that are the most harmful to them with some therapy, very few people are ever going to see a full recovery of their symptoms. It is going to be a constant struggle for these people and they are never going to be completely fixed. While things will get better for those who are associated with the person with the disorder, it is important for them to realize that the symptoms may never be gone.

While treatment can have some effectiveness at helping with the signs and symptoms of the personality disorder, many people do not get the help that they need at all. They think that the symptoms are not that bad and that they do not need help at all.

Many think that they will be able to work these things out without any help. But going in and getting the treatment that is needed is a big part of making sure that your symptoms are taken care of and that your quality of life is better.

It has been found that a lot of those who have the borderline personality disorder are also the ones who have other problems with their mental health. They may have issues such as substance abuse, eating disorders, and depression. Doing the proper treatment is going to help out with these issues as well.

How Others Can Help

Often, the loved ones of the person dealing with this personality disorder are distraught and do not know what to do. They want to be able to help this person, but they keep being turned away and shunned. One of the best things that you can do as a loved one for this person is be accepting. Acceptance that they have it and the willingness to help them out if needed is exactly what this person is going to need, even if it is hard for others to do this.

Many families do not want to accept that something is wrong within them or that the person they have known since they were a little kid has something wrong with them. But if you try to sweep it under the rug, the person you love who has the disorder is going to do the same and will never admit that they have a problem and get the help that they need.

Some of the ways that you can show your acceptance is to show that person lots of love and also take the time to learn as much as possible about this illness. Using this guidebook is a good way to get started as is talking to a specialist about the disorder. You also need to show some understanding. No matter how hard it may be, you must learn how to understand that any behavior that the person is showing, even if it is anger and hate that is coming to you, is not caused by this person but by the illness they have.

Next, you must know when it is time to get some help. This is a type of disorder that has the ability to make the person suicidal, violent, and angry. Often the disorder can go unnoticed for a long period of time so you are not going to have the luxury of waiting around to see how it goes once you find out. You need to take this seriously and call for the help that is needed if you think that this person is going to cause themselves of someone else some harm.

Also remember that the person with the disorder is not the only one who is going through all of this. This is a time that can be really hard on family members and they need to get the support they need in order to fully understand what is going on in the situation. Talk to the health department in your area to see if there are any support groups that are near for you to talk to. These groups will give you the information that you need in order to understand what is going on and to start taking things into your own hands.

As you can see, there is a lot that can go into this form of disease. It is not a simple one and those who are not close to the person who is suffering from borderline personality disorder may think that this person is just having a bad day or overreacting to the things that are going on around them. This is a disorder though that can take over the life of the person who is suffering and they may not see any way to get out of it. The right understanding and support from those they love, as well as some therapy, can help get them back on the right track.

One of the best ways that the person with this kind of disorder is going to get the help that they need is to get the support from those who they love. This can be hard for a lot of family members and there has bene evidence that shows that when family members find out about the disorder, they are less accepting of the condition as they were before. This is believed to be due to the fact that they know about the stigma that comes with this disorder and that they are given the information about it in the wrong way so that they are not able to understand it as well as they should.

If you know someone who has this disorder and who is trying to receive treatment, work to be there and show your support. This is going to help them to keep motivated on the right path to getting the treatment that they need to do better and it is the only way that they are going to receive the help that they need to get off this path and start living a happier and healthier life away from the disorder. Shaming them or being mad at them is not going to help anyone, even yourself, so it is best to get them the help and treatment that they need as well as the support ahead of time.

Chapter 2: Causes of Borderline Personality Disorder

It is always a good idea to learn some of the things that are going to be the cause of borderline personality disorder. This can sometimes help you to determine if someone has this kind of personality disorder. But unfortunately, it is not always possible to pinpoint the exact reason that someone is dealing with the disorder. Sometimes it will be one of the reasons or another and other times it will be several of them at the same time. Plus there is the added issue with the fact that just because a certain thing has occurred to someone or they are dealing with a particular issue that is listed here does not mean that they have borderline personality disorder.

As you can see, this is something that can be really confusing to know and understand. There is no straightforward way to determine what causes the personality disorder, but these causes can help to give a guess. Only a professional in the field will be able to go through the history of the patient, spend some time talking to them, and then determine if the causes are actually borderline personality disorder or something else.

As with many of the mental disorders that someone could have, the exact causes of this personality disorder are really complex and it has not been fully agreed upon what the exact causes are. There are some studies that show that this kind of personality disorder may be linked to post traumatic stress disorder. This does not mean that someone has to go into war or something that critical in order to get this disorder, but something may have caused severe stress to the person and that may be the link to them developing it.

Most researchers will agree that often a contributing factor to the personality disorder is that something traumatic happened in the persons' childhood, but there has not been much attention given in the past to see how the causal roles of other issues, which will be discussed in this chapter, would affect the issue as well. What this means is that it is very common for people who have been diagnosed with borderline personality disorder to have had some kind of trauma during their childhood, but usually this is also going to be coupled with something else, whether genetic, psychological issues, or another thing as well.

One thing that could be causing the issues with this personality disorder are some social factors. These would include the way that people will interact during their early years when it comes to other children, their friends and family. The child may also have something with psychological factors that get in the way of them developing the relationships that they should. These factors are usually going to include the temperament and personality which is shaped by their environment as well as any coping skills that they have learned in order to deal with the stresses in their lives.

What this all means is that there are a lot of different things that could be contributing to the personality disorder. No one is going to have the same beginning that gets them to dealing with this disorder, but it is important that they get the help that they need. Now let's spend some time looking at the different causes that may be to blame for the personality disorder.

Genetics

One of the main things that could be the cause of borderline personality disorder is genetics. It is estimated that at least 65 percent of the cases of this kind of personality disorder has some genes that were passed down that led them to have the disorder. What this number means is that 65 percent of the liability in the underlying disorder that is in the population can be explained by the genetic differences.

This can be a really difficult thing to understand. You may not have anyone in your family who has the disorder and it may never happen to anyone else in your family. What this means is that some of the genes in your body have made it more likely that you will develop the personality issues that come from this disorder.

The effect of the genes on this and other disorders have been done quite a bit in the past with the use of twins. While these can provide some powerful insights into the way that genes would work, it is important to remember that when it comes to twins, they are going to have a lot of the same environmental factors so they can have the same issues just because they live in the same environment rather than because of the genes. This is why it is often easier to determine what can happen if researchers are able to find twins who were separated at birth from adoption or other circumstances.

In the Netherlands, there was a study with families of twins. In this study, there were 711 sibling pairs and 561 parents and all of them were examined in order to identify where the genetic traits were located that would influence borderline personality disorder occurring. Researchers for this project found that the material in the genes that was associated with this personality disorder is found on the chromosome nine. Studies also concluded that about 42 percent of this variation of the disorder futures would be attributed to different genetics while the rest of it would be attributed to environmental influences.

This means that while genes can be partially to blame for the issue with this disorder, it is possible for a person to have the right genetic factors without ever developing the disorder at all. It seems that the environmental factors need to be present, as they are more crucial to the issue, in order to see the disorder develop in anyone.

Brain Abnormalities

The next thing that we will look at that may cause the disorder are issues that come in the brain. There are several studies that were done that did neuroimaging of those with this disorder. These studies show that those who have the disorder have reductions in the regions of their brains that are in charge of the responses for emotions and stress, affect the hippocampus, and amygdala, and even the orbitofrontal cortex. There are some smaller studies that did more of this and found that some other areas of the brain that influenced the emotions that the person has.

This section will look at some of the areas of the brain that can be affected in the person who is suffering from this kind of disorder.

Hippocampus

The hippocampus is one area of the brain that tends to look smaller in those who are dealing with borderline personality disorder. This is the same area that is going to be smaller in those who are going through post-traumatic stress disorder which is why the two issues are usually linked together. However, there are also other parts of the brain that are affected, which are not affected in PTSD, which means that this cannot be the only cause of the disorder.

Amygdala

Another area of the brain that is smaller as well as more active in those who are suffering from the disorder is the amygdala. This is something that is going to be found in those who are going through obsessive compulsive disorder so this may be another thing that those with the personality disorder are dealing with as well.

There has been some studies done on this and one of them found that when someone who is dealing with this disorder is experiencing or viewing some negative emotions, they are going to have some really strong activity in their left amygdala that is not usual in most people. Since the amygdala is the area that is going to generate all of the emotions of the person, this is including all of the negative emotions, this strong activity might be the explanation of why a person with the disorder has such a long time and such intense emotions when it comes to shame, anger, sadness, and fear. This could also be the explanation for why they are so sensitive compared to the situation and how others would react as well.

Prefrontal cortex

This is an area of the brain that is going to be much less active in those who are suffering from this kind of personality disorder. This is going to be extra apparent when the person is recalling any memories of being abandoned. This little activity is going to occur in the right side on the anterior cingulate. Given the role that it has in regulating the amount of arousal that they will get in their emotions when something occurs. This inactivity may be the explanation for why it is difficult for a person with this disorder to regular their own emotions as well as the responses that they have to stress.

What this means is that because they are not getting the activity that is needed in the prefrontal cortex they are not able to keep their emotions in check and so they are going to let them go all over the place. This is one of the reasons why medication is often needed to help with this personality disorder. It allows them to get the parts of the brain working again so that they can actually start to deal with their emotions in a healthy way.

Hypothalamic, pituitary, adrenal axis

This is a long name for a part of the brain that is going to regulate the amount of cortisol that is produced. This is a chemical that is released in order to help the person deal with the stresses that they are feeling. Cortisol production is often going to be much higher in those who are dealing with this personality disorder, meaning that this area of the brain is really hyperactive. This is going to cause the person to experience a lot more biological stress than other people would which is an explanation for why they are more likely to get irritated over little things.

One of the reasons that this area may be more active is because it will increase the cortisol production is traumatic experiences. This is why many of those who are suffering from this kind of personality disorder are dealing with this since they dealt with some kind of trauma when they were younger.

Another thing that might be causing it is their disorder is that when they have the heightened sensitivity to different stresses in their lives, the increase in the cortisol is going to make those who are already dealing with this disorder to be predisposed to experiencing childhood stresses and having them be stressful.

This increase in the cortisol production is often associated with a higher risk of the suicidal behavior that is found in people, whether they are going through this disorder or not.

Neurobiological Factors

The next issue that could be causing someone to have this kind of disorder would be neurobiological factors. These will be discussed in more details below.

Estrogen

The differences that can come during a woman's estrogen cycle can sometimes be the reason that the symptoms of this disorder are going to show up in females. There was a study done in 2003 that showed that the symptoms of borderline personality disorder in women were able to be predicted based on the levels of estrogen and how much they changed throughout the menstrual cycle. This is an effect that was still significant when the results became more controlled for the general increase in the negative effects.

The symptoms that would be experienced due to the levels of estrogen being disturbed are sometimes misdiagnosed as this kind of personality disorder though so it is important to be careful when doing this. Some of the symptoms that could go with this disorder are also going to be found just in PMS as well as PMDD so just because a woman is acting a bit moody does not mean that she has a personality disorder. Some examples of the symptoms that can be mistaken would include depression and mood swings that are severe.

In those who do have this kind of personality disorder, those who were going through psychotic episodes could be treated with some estrogen and there would be a lot of improvement. But it is important to note that this treatment is not going to be prescribed to women who have endometriosis because the estrogen is going to worsen this condition. If the estrogen is the issue with women and this disorder, any drugs that are used to stabilize the mood are not going to help. The diagnosis needs to be studied by a professional and correct diagnosed before knowing whether estrogen treatments are the right course of action or if they are safe.

Other Issues

Estrogen is not the only thing that could be causing the issue which is shown by the fact that men can also have this kind of disorder. There has been studies that show a strong correlation that occurs between child abuse and the development of this personality disorder. Many individuals who are suffering from it will be able to report that they have a history of neglect and abuse when they were a small child. Patients who have this disorder may have a higher likelihood of being sexually, physically, emotionally, or verbally abused when they were younger and this is usually abuse that has been done by a caretaker of some kind; the gender was not just male or female since it could have been either depending on the case. There is also a high rate of the person with the disorder losing a caregiver they were close to as a child and incest.

Next, those with this kind of disorder are much likely to have had a caregiver in their past, regardless of the sex, deny that they had any feelings or thoughts that were valid. These caregivers also would have failed to provide any of the protections that their child needed and often they would have neglected the physical care that was due to the child. Parents of each sex would also be reported as withdrawn from their children emotionally and may have been inconsistent with the way that they were treating the child.

In addition, the women who had this kind of disorder would report that in their past they were neglected by their female caregiver while being abused by the male caregiver and then they would experience sexual abuse by someone who was not their caregiver. Because of these findings, it is often suggested that children that are mistreated during their childhood and are dealing with issues with attachment may eventually go on to develop this kind of personality disorder.

It is important to remember though that just because a child experiences some trauma when they were a child it does not mean that they are going to automatically suffer from this kind of personality disorder. Rather, the trauma is a contributing factor, but other things are going to need to be in place. For example, the children may have been put through these horrible experiences because the parent was dealing with the disorder in their genes and then it was passed down to the child. The trauma is only going to result in the person developing this disorder if other things are present and if they are predisposed to it in the first place.

Developmental Factors

While some sufferers of this disorder are going to undergo childhood sexual abuse, this is not always a good way to determine who has or is going to develop borderline personality disorder. Often the reactivity and intensity of the person to negative emotions are going to be a better way to predict the symptoms of this disorder much better. This finding as well as the differences to the structure of the brain in these people and the issue with some patients not having any traumatic history in their path sometimes suggests that the disorder is somewhat distinct form PTSD. While they share some similarities, they are not one and the same. This is why researchers began to do some examining on different developmental causes that will affect who suffers from this disorder.

Some newer research that was published in 2013 through the University of Toronto has found that there are two patterns that can apply to brain activity that may be the underlying reason that there are issues with regulating the emotions; something that is very common with this disorder. While this goes into a lot of details about how the brain in a person with this disorder is working, it basically states that those who are dealing with the borderline personality disorder are basically set up by the brains in order to have emotional lives that are stormy. This does not mean that their lives are really that unproductive or unhappy, but since the different regions of the brain are over or under producing, they are going to seem like they are way more emotional than they should be.

This shows that many of the issues are in the brain. The brain is not working properly so the patient is not being fed the right kind of information or given the chance to deal with the situation or the emotions in a reasonable way. Since this is occurring, they are going to feel more intense emotions that are out of context and to them there is no negotiating to see if someone is good or bad because their brain just flips without much decision making. This is why it is so hard to treat those with this disorder; they are dealing with improper working of their brains and it can take years to get it rewired to work properly.

Other Factors

While the above factors are often the first ones that are going to be looked for when it comes to a person who is dealing with borderline personality disorder, there are a lot of other factors that will need to be taken into consideration. Some of these will be discussed a bit more below.

Executive function

While it is true that a sensitivity to rejection is high in someone who has really strong symptoms of this disorder, the executive functions of the brain appear to be the things that mediate the relationships between the two. This means that there are a group of processes that will include problem solving, attention, working memory, and planning and they may be the thing that allows rejection sensitivity to impact the symptoms of this personality disorder.

There was a study done in 2008 which found that this relationship between the symptoms of this disorder and the sensitivity the person had to rejection were much stronger when their executive function was going the opposite way and was lower.

Of course, this also means that when the executive function worked at a higher rate, the symptoms would be much weaker. What this suggests is that having a higher executive function would possibly be able to help people who had a high level of symptoms with this disorder.

Also, another study done in 2012 say that when there were issues with the working memory, there might be a likelihood that the person would be more impulsive when they were also suffering from the disorder. This could explain why many people who are dealing with borderline personality disorder were so interested in being impulsive and doing other activities that they shouldn't.

Family environment

In some of the cases of borderline personality disorder, the person who is dealing with this disorder is going to have a few family environment issues that were able to cause the disorder. This is often in the form of sexual abuse. It is important to realize though that just because sexual abuse occurred does not mean that someone is going to develop this disorder and not all of the people who get this disorder will have been sexually abused. What this does mean is that there is a higher percentage of those who were sexually abused or harmed during their childhood who later develop this kind of disorder.

Often a family environment that is unstable is able to predict whether this disorder is going to develop or not. The unstable environment increases the likelihood that the person is going to suffer from the disorder while a stable environment is going to show a lower risk. One explanation for why this might be so is because the stable environment can help as a bugger against the disorder developing even if some other risk factors are present.

Thought Suppression

There was a study done in 2005 which showed that though suppression may have been a connection between the symptoms of this disorder and emotional vulnerability. Basically the thought suppression is going to be the action of the person to attempt to avoid having certain thoughts even if they might be considered natural. There was also a study found later on that showed that this relationship is not necessarily mediated through this suppression, but that it could help lead to the symptoms of this disorder.

What this means is that if the person is suppressing some of the emotions that they are feeling, it could eventually lead them to this disorder. They might be holding the emotions down so deep and not know what to do with them. The more emotions they stuff down deep, the less that they are able to understand about the rest of the world and the less they will be able to properly handle the emotions that they are feeling. This can result in a lot of complexities for the person and it can make things difficult for them to figure out.

As you can see from this, there is not just one situation that is going to cause the person to suffer from borderline personality disorder. It is usually a combination of things that will get it all to start and it can sometimes be a really deep rooted issue. When you start to see the more complexities that come with the issue, you can start to understand why so much therapy and work is needed in order to have any hopes of doing a good job with the recovery phase, if it even get to that point.

Chapter 3: Signs and Symptoms of Recognizing Borderline Personality Disorder

It is important that you are able to recognize the signs of borderline personality disorder so that the person who is suffering from it, whether it is you or someone else, is able to get the help that they need as soon as possible. It is really difficult to determine if someone has personality disorder like this one because they are often going to keep others far away. Those around them will just assume that the mood swings are because of a long day and they will often just think that the person has friends and family in another aspect of their lives rather than that the person is all on their own.

Recognizing some of the symptoms of personality disorder can really make it easier to help the person when they need it. We will get into more details about some of the specifics of these signs and symptoms, but basically, some of the symptoms you may notice with someone with borderline personality disorder include:

- Lots of other mental health issues such as rage, substance abuse, anger, anxiety, and depression. You will find that when they are dealing with the borderline personality disorder, these underlying causes will sometimes make things a lot worse and without treating the depression or anger or other issue, they are not going to have a chance of getting better.

- Impulsivity—they just want to get a thrill ride out of their lives and so they are going to do something that is fun and has a lot of risk. This is a way for them to get a little relief from their emotions, which they cannot control, for just a bit of time. The problem comes after the thrill is done thought. They are going to start feeling like they did something wrong and the guilt and worry are going to be worse than in the beginning. This can turn into a vicious cycle of trying to feel better without any results.

- Self-damaging behavior—this might include things like cutting or burning themselves and could even include substance abuse. This is going to happen because the person with this disorder is going to put all of their feelings internally. They rarely if ever will hurt other people when they are upset or angry and

74

instead they will do it to themselves. They may also do this because they do not think that they are worth anything and so

- Concerns about being abandoned—people with this kind of personality disorder are always worried about being abandoned. Often this is their own doing though; they might get mad at the people who are trying to get close to them and cause them to go away or they may figure that they do not want to get hurt so they do not let anyone in.

- Unstable self-esteem and relationships— pretty much, these kinds of people do not have any relationships and if they do, the relationships are not very strong and are not going to hurt this person if they end. They also have very low self-esteem.

- Intense emotions that cannot be controlled— the person with borderline personality disorder is going to have a lot of issues with their emotions and they will not know how to control these emotions. Think about a young kid and how they are able to go back and forth between emotions in no time because they do not know the first thing about controlling them. This is the same thing that occurs with someone with this disorder.

- A sense of identity that is very disturbed—they do not know who they are or what their purpose is. They may think that everyone hates them mostly because they do not understand how things work.

- Chaos in their relationships—any relationships that are around are going to be a mess and probably will not last very long. For the most part, those who have this disorder are not going to have relationships that are good at all. They will have one for a short time that might be intense, but any little thing could set them off and they will get out of the relationship in no time. This is hard for others to be close to them because of this difficulty with their emotions.

These are just a few of the symptoms and signs that you will need to watch out for when it comes to dealing with someone with personality disorder. It is important to know all of these to determine if someone is going through this and needs some help. Some of the more intense side effects will be discussed in the following sections.

Emotional Symptoms

Let's take some time to look at the emotional symptoms that a person with this kind of disorder may have. People who are suffering from borderline personality disorder are the ones that are going to feel their emotions more than the others around them. They may feel them for a longer period of time, most deeply, and even more easily than other do. Also, these emotions are going to persist and come back over and over again. You may notice that the event to disturb them happened weeks ago, but the person is still suffering from some intense emotions because it will take them quite some time in order to get back to their emotional baseline and be stable again.

The emotions can go from one end of the spectrum to the other and they are not always about being sad, upset, or angry. Some people with this kind of disorder may be loving, joyful, idealistic, and enthusiastic, but at some times these may be to the extreme. Just because they can feel these positive emotions to an extreme does not mean that they are not going to become overwhelmed by all of the negative emotions that are surrounding them as well. For example, instead of feeling just sadness over an event they may feel some intense grief. They could feel humiliation and shame rather than just being a little embarrassed at a situation. Rage is often shown instead of annoyance and panic will show whenever they are nervous.

Often, these emotions are not totally out of the blue. There may be something that caused an emotion in the first place, but since these people are not able to recognize and control their emotions, the emotion is going to be blown way out of proportion. For example, instead of just being a bit embarrassed because you tripped going up on stage a bit, the person will feel like it is the end of the world and that everyone is laughing at them all of the time. In addition, instead of being just sad that their favorite show is over, they may hold onto this as intense grief for weeks to come.

People with this disorder are going to be really sensitive to what they perceive as their own failure, isolation, criticism, and being rejected. This is the person who at work you are just giving a suggestion to make things easier, not even really telling them they did anything wrong, and instead of taking it in stride and recognizing you are trying to help, they will overreact and think that you are telling them they have failed and are a horrible person. The emotion will go way out of proportion and they may hold onto this idea for a long period of time. The fact that they refuse to work with you and think that you are now against them is going to enhance their feeling of isolation because you really are not going to want to have anything to do with them.

Often the issues with them exhibiting suicidal behavior or causing themselves injury is due to the fact that the person with the disorder does not have any other way to cope with the things that are going on around them. They do not know that therapy, writing things in a diary, talking to others, or even living a healthy lifestyle will be able to help them to get through these emotions in a much safer and healthier way. Since they do not know this and their emotions are all over the place, they may feel like these two things are the only options that are available to them.

In some cases, the person with this disorder is going to be aware that their emotions are way off the grid and not acceptable to others, but they do not know how to control or regular these emotions. They then figure out that the best idea is to shut the emotions down all of the way. This is actually the part where a lot of people find out about the person suffering from borderline personality disorder since the negative emotions are going to alert others of the problem and they are going to work in order to address it.

Of course, there are times when a person with this kind of disorder is going to feel some intense joy in their lives, but since they are more prone to the feelings of dysphoria, or feelings of emotional and mental distress, this joy may not show itself very much. The dysphoria can make the situation worse because it heightens a lot of the issues that were already present in this person and makes them more pronounced. Those who are suffering from dysphoria may also experience feelings of being a victim, feeling of lacking an identity or being fragmented, being destructive to either themselves or to others, and going through extreme emotions.

While the person with this disorder is going to have emotional changeability, it is not the same as some others who are going through mood swings. Often these kinds of things imply that the person is going back and forth between being happy and then being sad. But with this kind of person, it often means that they are going to vary between anxiety and anger and then between anxiety and depression. While feelings of being happy can come about at times, usually the person is going to swing back and forth between these more negative feelings.

Behavior Symptoms

For those who are dealing with this disorder, it is not uncommon to have impulsive behavior. This would include things like reckless driving, reckless spending, having sex with multiple partners without using protection, eating disorders, alcohol abuse, and substance abuse. In addition, the impulsive behavior can start to go to other parts of the persons like such as self-injury, running away, and leaving out on relationships and jobs.

You may be wondering why a person with this kind of disorder would have anything to do with behavior of this kind. Basically it is a way for them to get some relief from the pain they are feeling from the emotions. These people are not able to control the emotions that they are feeling and often they will not understand why they are feeling emotions that are so intense. When they do the impulsive behavior, it gives them a nice rush, a moment of feeling better, and they begin to crave that moment in order to get a break from the crazy emotions that are boiling up in them.

It is important to note that even though this is used as a method of escape, in the long term these people are going to end up feeling more pain from their actions because they feel guilty and shameful for participating in them. This is a horrible cycle that is just going to make the person feel so much worse in the long run. In some cases, it may go on so long though that the impulsive behavior is done without thought when some kind of emotional pain comes to the person.

Self-harm

Many of those who are suffering from borderline personality disorder are going to have some issues with harming themselves or with suicidal behavior. In fact, this is one of the main criteria that will be used in helping to determine if a person actually has this kind of disorder or not. Management and then the subsequent recovery of this kind of behavior is going to be challenging and complex. There is always going to be a risk of suicide for the whole life of this person and the risk is somewhere between 3 percent and ten percent. While this might not be a high number of people who have committed suicide, many others with this condition will have thought about it in the past and may have attempted but did not succeed. There is also evidence that shows that men who are diagnosed with this condition are about twice as likely as women to commit suicide when they are diagnosed. There has also been some thoughts that many of the men who are thought to randomly commit suicide may have borderline personality disorder but they were not diagnosed.

Even if the person is not considering suicide or having these kinds of thoughts, it is still pretty common that they are going to perform some kind of self-injury to themselves. The reasons for the injuries are often different than the reasons for attempting suicide in most people. The reason for attempting to cause harm to themselves without trying to perform suicide are often to distract someone from their emotional pain, trying to generate normal feelings when they are feeling disassociated, as a form of punishment, and a way to express anger.

In contrast, when the person tries to commit suicide, they are showing thoughts that they believe that others would be better without them once the suicide is done. Both of these kinds of injuries are going to be the response of the person who is going through these negative emotions. They think that the abuse is going to let them feel normal or bring them back to reality and make things better, even though this is not the case.

One thing to note is that most of the people who have this disorder are usually not going to be able to cause any physical harm to those around them. Often this kind of personality disorder is going to be shown in the wrong light and many think that they are a bit crazy and could cause harm to those around them. Since most of those with this disorder have had abuse when they were younger, they are very against hurting others and any of the harm that they are going to do will be done to themselves rather to anyone else.

Interpersonal Relationships

Those who are dealing with this kind of disorder are often going to be really sensitive to the ways that others may be treating them. They may feel really intense gratitude and joy when they think that someone is treating them with a lot of kindness. On the other hand, they may feel some intense anger and sadness when they feel that someone else is criticizing or making them feel hurt. The feelings that they have about others is going to shift from one day or another and it will depend on the way that the person treats them, or at least the way that the person perceives they are being treated. They will often be worried about losing those they trust and they do not want to feel like they are going down in esteem from someone else.

This is a phenomenon that is known as black and white thinking or splitting and is going to include having a shift from idealizing others to devaluing them. The person does not see that things come in different colors and will only see them in black and white. For example, they may like someone at one moment and then may not like them or want anything to do with them because that person gave them a little criticism or didn't have enough time for them one time.

When this kind of thing is combined with devaluation, idealization, and the many mood disturbances that come with this disorder means that it is really hard for the person to have any relationships whether it is with their coworkers, friends, and family. Their own personal self-image is going to change from positive to negative very rapidly which can make them even more difficult to do deal with.

This can be really hard for the person who is suffering from the disorder because they really want to have some intimacy with those around them. Because they want the intimacy and are not getting it, they are more likely to be preoccupied with the attachment patterns in their relationships, they will feel insecure, and they may avoid other people. They may also see the world as a malevolent and dangerous place because they are not able to find the intimacy that they desire. The issue here is that they are often the ones who are keeping others at bay, even if someone wants to try and get with them.

In some cases of borderline personality disorder, the person may find that manipulation is the only way they are able to get the nurturing and intimacy that they would like. It is not that they want to be in control of the people who are near them though, like what is found in other mental illnesses. Rather, it is about trying to get someone to like them and they are not sure how else to do this process.

Sense of Self

One of the more noticeable things that others will say about someone who has this disorder. People with this disorder are going to have some trouble seeing who they are and they may see themselves as something much less. While others are going to see them as a great person who has gotten a lot of accomplishments and would be there to help anyone who needed it, the person is going to see themselves as worthless and someone that no one else would want to hang out with.

Often, these kinds of people are going to have a lot of difficulties with understanding that they have value and that others do really enjoy them when their emotions are not all over the place. In addition, they may often be unsure about their log terms goals whether it is for their life, jobs, or even relationships. This whole thing with not knowing who they are or the things that they value can make them feel more empty and lost.

Everyone has a time in their lives when they are going to feel like they are not sure of the goals that they want to reach in their lives. They may have just gotten out of school and were not able to get the job that they always wanted. Other times they may be worried about if they will be able to pay a bill or something else. It is normal to have times when the future is not so certain. But the person with this disorder is going to feel this way all of the time. They never have a plan for their life and they are always going to feel like they have no idea where they should be going.

It is pretty easy to tell if someone is having too much issues with their sense of self. These are usually people who are really good at what they can do, who might be the most loving and fun people to be around when they are dealing with their emotions the correct way, and they can be just as talented as others. But despite all of this, they are going to be very unsure of themselves and feel like they are not able to do anything write. They are going to go around believing that no one could possibly like them no matter what, and these feelings are not going to be because they feel like this is the way that they can get attention. Instead, they are doing it because they actually feel this way and nothing you do will convince them that this is the wrong way to think about themselves.

Cognitions

Finally, there are also going to be some cognition differences that occur in the person who is suffering from borderline personality disorder. Often the really intense emotions that these people will experience will make it really difficult for them to be able to control their attention and their focus. Often you will see that they are not able to concentrate on something for very long and they may spend a lot of time dissociating or zoning out during the day. Dissociation is an occurrence that is a response in some people when they are experiencing a somewhat painful event; or at least experiencing something that will make them remember that painful event.

During dissociation, the mind is going to automatically redirect the person's attention away from the painful event in order to protect them and make sure that some unwanted impulses do not happen. Although this is technically a way for the mind to block out these painful and intense emotions in order to provide some relief, in some cases it can block out even the good feelings that a person is experiencing and makes the person feel more numb.

Those with this kind of disorder is going to find that it is impossible to make decisions because they do not have these normal emotions.

In some cases, it might be possible for an outsider to notice when the person with the disorder is dissociation, because the vocal and facial expressions can become expressionless or they may become flat and they will look distracted. Then again, there are times when it is impossible to tell when someone is going through dissociation at all.

This is a complex way of saying that the person with the disorder is not able to feel the emotions that are around them properly because their brains are not letting them. As mentioned before, a lot of the people who are dealing with this disorder have had something that was traumatic in their childhood. This could have been abuse, neglect, or the loss of someone who was close to them. Because of this bad experience, the person is going through dissociation about that event and if something reminds them of the event, they will go through the dissociation again.

While this might seem like it is a good way to protect the person, and most of the time when the process occurs that is exactly what is happening, when dissociation occurs too often, the person is going to be blocking out a lot of emotions that are a part of their daily life. They are going to miss out on joy, friendships, love, and happiness, as well as some of the bad things, because their mind is still trying to protect them and get them away from a situation that it thinks is harmful.

This could be used to describe why the person with borderline personality disorder reacts in this way. They are missing out on some of the emotions that are important to their lives and so they are not getting the full experience that is needed. Without that, they are not able to make the right decisions in order to make friends, get things done, or even think about their futures. They do not realize they are missing out on these emotions though so to them they are not seeing a problem at all.

Also, if the brain is forcing the person to go through dissociation when emotions start to come up, how is that person supposed to learn how to control all of their emotions? They might have these emotions come up randomly and they have to try and deal with them while other times the brain my try to take over instead. This is why many of those with this disorder are going to have a lot of trouble handling their emotions simply because they might not be as used to them as they should be.

Often therapy will look at this dissociation to figure out if it might be the issue behind some of the behavioral and emotional problems of this person. If the dissociation can be helped out, the person is going to be able to start learning about all of the emotions and learning how to deal with them rather than hiding. This process is going to be a slow one, but over time, they will learn what is going to work and that things are not as black and white as they have been used to seeing.

One of the only ways that you are going to be able to get help for this disorder is to get a diagnosis and treatment from a professional. The success rate for those who are able to go into treatment and stay for the required amount of time is the majority so it is really worth your time to go in and get the help. Asking for help can be difficult, but it is the only way to get control over the issue and get the best help possible. A professional will be able to diagnose this and make sure that the right questions and treatment are being offered to each client to get them to feel better.

These are just a few of the signs and symptoms of borderline personality disorder. It is important to understand these so that you are able to get the person the help that they need in order to stay healthy and get through the issues. Many people do not understand what is going on with this disorder so they will simply say that the person is crazy and should just get over it. But understanding where all of the behaviors and actions are coming from helps to show that the person is not actually able to control

the way that they are acting and behaving.

Chapter 4: Diagnosis of the Disorder

One of the hardest things to do with this kind of disorder is to diagnose it. Most of the people who have it are not going to want to have anything to do with the doctor or psychiatrist who is trying to help them out and so they are going to ignore them and not take the help. Often it is going to take family members to see the issue and initiate the help that is needed before the person with the disorder is going to get the help. They are not going to go in on their own because they are not going to see that they have any issues at all.

Once you can get the person with the disorder to come into the door, the diagnosis of this disorder is going to be based on the assessment that is done in the clinic by a professional of mental health. The best way to do this is to present the different criteria of the disorder to the patient, these criteria are listed above, and ask them if they think that any of these describe them. This is going to get the participant involved in the cure, making it more likely to work. Plus, a doctor is usually not going to have enough time or outside experience with the patient in order to determine on their own if the characteristics are there and this can provide them with a usually truthful means of getting to it.

When you allow the person who has this kind of disorder to actively help with the diagnosis, they are going to be more willing to get the help that the professional is going to get them. There are some clinicians though who decide that it is best to not tell their patients that they have this diagnosis because they believe that it is full of stigma and the person will be against the treatment because they may have heard in the past that this is an untreatable disorder. While this is one way to go, there is a lot of research to show that the person suffering from the disease should know about it in order to get the most effective treatment that is possible.

During this evaluation, the patient is going to be asked a lot of questions about their symptoms including when they began and how severe they were. The might also be asked some questions that relate to how these symptoms are impacting their life. Some of the issues that the doctor is going to take special notes about would be any thoughts that are about harming others, experiences with doing self-harm, and any thoughts of suicide that the person has.

The diagnosis is going to be based on what the patient has been reporting at sessions as well as what the doctor has been able to observe in their short time. These two things are usually going to be able to combine to give a good outlook on what is going on. There are a few other tests that can be done to help determine if borderline personality disorder is present in the person. Sometimes some laboratory tests or a physical exam are going to be done in order to help rule out some of the other things that might trigger these symptoms, such as the person abusing substances or a thyroid condition; both of which could cause some of the same behaviors as what is find in borderline personality disorder.

Once the disorder has been determined and diagnosed in a patient, it is time to get to work with giving them the treatment that they need to stay healthy and get their lives back. While this is going to be a lot of work and will take some time, it is something that must be done if the person wants to get their life back and be much happier. Here is some more information about how the disorder could be diagnosed and how the person should get the help that they need to start feeling better in no time.

International Classifications

There are a few classifications that you will be able to find that are used internationally to help make the diagnosis. These classifications can be nice because they allow the clinician to be able to do the diagnosis without having to go on their own personal beliefs and can keep everything organized and the same throughout. The idea of borderline personality disorder, is one that is recognized by the World

Health Organization. It is then divided into two other categories which will be discussed a bit below.

Impulsive Type

The first kind of category that is recognized in this is the impulsive type. Out of the things that are discussed below, at least three of them need to be present in order to diagnose someone with this category of the disorder.

1. A marked tendency to get out of control or to act out. This is going to happen unexpectedly and will not be due to someone causing the issue or forcing them to act out. Often the act is going to be done by the person without them worrying or even thinking about the

consequences that could happen with their action. This is just something that they are going to do, perhaps over a slight disagreement or other issue, that should not have been that big of a deal but which was turned into one.

2. A marked tendency of the sufferer to get into behavior that is considered quarrelsome and they are going to have a lot of conflicts with the others around them. This is especially going to be true with impulsive acts that have been criticized or thwarted. This is a person who is routinely getting into fights with others around them and who see any little slight as an excuse to get in a big fight together.

3. A liability to having strong outbursts when it comes to violence or anger. Not only are they having these issues, but they do not have the ability that is needed in order to control the

explosions or other issues that come up. They will seem very angry but they will also seem like they do not have the means to come back down and be calm again even if they had wanted.

4. These people are also going to have some difficulty in staying with their course of action if they are not able to get a reward right away. They may have been really interested in doing it, but when it did not provide the immediate reward that they were looking for, they most likely became upset and angry and so decided to just give up on it. This is something that would happen quite often and the person would only stick with things they know they can finish and be rewarded with.

5. These people will often have capricious and unstable moods that can change almost

without any warning. It might be hard to keep up with these kinds of people.

These are the five criteria that will often be found in someone who is dealing with the impulsive kind of this disorder. You are going to notice that they are going to do things often without any thought to what they are doing or what is going to happen when they are done, and this can be a dangerous thing. For a person to be diagnosed with this kind of disorder, they are going to need to have at least three of the things mentioned above present when they talk to their therapist in the office.

Borderline Type

Next comes the borderline type. This one is going to be a little bit different. This is going to take a bit from the list above and then adds in a bit from the list that is going to be presented below. You will need to have a minimum of three of those symptoms that are found for the impulsive type present as well as a minimum of 2 of the ones below in order to get a diagnosis of this category. Some of the things to look for include:

1. A person with this type would often have some uncertainty and disturbances in their self-image as well as their internal preferences and their aims in life. They do not think that they are worth much and even though they crave interaction with others, they are not sure why these others would want to have anything to do with them. They may wonder around a lot looking confused because they do not know who they are, what

they should do with their lives, or what is to become of them.

2. They might also have a higher liability to get involved in relationships that are often unstable and intense. This might include those whirlwind relationships where they meet and get married in just a few short months, but it does not have to be this severe either in order to fit. Since the relationship is so unstable it is not going to last and since it was intense, it is likely to cause a sort of emotional crisis in the person who is suffering from the disorder.

3. These people are going to show really excessive efforts to never become abandoned. They are scared that one day they will wake up and not have anyone around to be their friends or to help them out when they need. This is further complicated by the fact that

they are pushing others away and are not very good at seeing other's points of view. They are going to work almost obsessively to make sure that others do not leave them alone so that they can always have the help and companionship that they are looking for.

4. They are also going to have frequent threats as well as acts of self-harm. This is often not in an attempt to get someone to act the way that they would like or to change the feelings of someone else. This is more of something that they do in the hopes of getting their own emotions in check. They are going to have a lot of trouble with their own emotions and since they are not able to keep them under control, they may turn to self-harm in the hopes of getting some relief.

5. Frequent feelings that surround them of emptiness. Because they do not have any

plans for their future or for the things that they want to do in their lives, they are going to feel empty. They do not have any goals or long term plans, so often they are just going to wander around and hope that things work out the best. This can lead to a life that is pretty empty.

6. They are going to often demonstrate behavior that is impulsive. This is going to include things such as substance abuse and speeding. The idea behind doing these things is because it gives the sufferer a bit of a break for the bad feelings or uncontrolled emotions that they are going through so that they can just feel better for a bit. The issue comes when the person begins to feel a bit guilty about their behavior and so they will feel even worse than they did before.

As mentioned before, there needs to be quite a few things that are present before someone is going to be diagnosed with this form of the disorder. But those who meet these requirements should get the help that they need as soon as possible.

Millon's Subtypes

First we are going to take a look at the different subtypes that are used when it comes to borderline personality disorder. Theodore Millon has in the past proposed that there are four different subtypes when it comes to borderline personality disorder. Within these different categories, a person who has this disorder is going to exhibit usually one of more of the following things (these include the subtypes of the person with borderline personality disorder as well as the features that come with it):

- Discouraged—this subtype is also going to include the features of someone who is avoidant. You will find that a person who fits into this category is powerless, helpless, depressed, feels like there is no hope for them or their live, feels like they are in a constant jeopardy and vulnerable, humble, loyal, submissive, and pliant.

- Petulant—this category is also going to include the features of someone who is very negative about the thing that are going on around them. You will find that a person who fits into this category is quickly disillusioned and that they can be slighted at a moment's notice, resentful, pessimistic, sullen, defiant and really stubborn to get along with, restless, impatient, and very negative about everything.

- Impulsive—this category is also going to include the features of someone who is very antisocial and does not want to be around others. Some of the features that you will find in a person who suffers from this include someone who is potentially suicidal, someone who is irritable, gloomy, and can become agitated on occasion. These people are going to be fearful of losing things and are frenetic, distractible, flighty, superficial, and capricious.

- Self-destructive—this category is also going to include the features of someone is very masochistic or depressive. They are going to be really moody and high strung and these are going to show up more and more over time, they may think at times about suicide as an option are many of their positive features are going to begin to deteriorate. They are deferential, conforming, and angry over little things, and will turn inwards to themselves rather than making friends.

It is possible for someone to fit into more than one of these categories and have this kind of disorder, but this kind of helps to divide out the different symptoms and make them make a bit more sense for those who are learning about them or diagnosing them.

The Conclusion

While there are a variety of different thoughts that come with this disorder, they all are pretty much going to work together in order to summarize what is going on with this disorder. It is not a simple one and there is not necessarily one definition that is going to be able to describe what is going on for each case. While some cases are going to have abuse in the past of the sufferer, not all of the cases will have had abuse and even if a person was abused in the past it does not mean that they are going to get this disorder. There are a lot of things that need to be in place for this issue to show up and it is complicated to take control of.

Even those who are trained to deal with this kind of condition are going to find that sometimes it is hard to diagnose it as the right personality disorder and sometimes it can be given the wrong diagnosis. This can be harmful to the sufferer because they are not going to be getting the help that they need at the right time. But the definitions that are given above are able to give a good starting point, as well as some experience and training, will help the professional to give the right diagnosis so the sufferer can get the help that they need.

Family Members

Even the way that the person with the disorder is treating the others who are around them can be a way of diagnosing them. People who have this disorder are going to be much more prone to disliking their family members and they are often going to be angry at these same people. Often the person with the disorder is going to work in order to alienate themselves from the family because they are mad over some little slight or they are worried that the family members are going to become to see a problem. Often the family members are going to feel a bit helpless and angry about the way that they are relating with this person and may wonder what they can do in order to make things right again.

There was a study done in 2003 that found that the thoughts of the family members would change once they found out that the behavior was for a reason. In most cases, the anger and hurt towards the person with the disorder would go up once their family members began to understand what is going on. While this would not seem like something that would happen, it is often believed that these feelings are occurring because the family is being given the wrong kind of information about the disorder so they are blaming the person rather than the issue at hand.

The best way for family members to be able to help out the one that they love is to learn as much as possible about the disorder. It is easy to start looking through books and watching shows about the disorder and while this might be a good place to start in some cases, you will find that it is often the wrong information. Get out there and find the information that is the right information and this is going to help make more sense out of what you are seeing with your loved one.

This is going to be just as difficult for members of the family to handle as it is for the person who is going through the issue. They are the ones who have been emotionally harmed by their loved one not wanting to have anything to do with them. It is important that the family gets the therapy and help that they need in order to feel better about the situation.

Understanding the whole situation and how it is affecting the family and the sufferer can make it easier to get through the whole situation together.

Adolescence

The on set of these symptoms of the disorder are usually going to happen sometime in adolescence or in young adulthood. In some cases, it is possible for the symptoms to occur in children, but this is not as prevalent. Symptoms that occur among a teenager is going to predict if borderline personality disorder is going to occur in their adult life. Some of the symptoms that can be present include severe shame, attempts to get in an exclusive relationship that often will not work out, self-injury that is not committing suicide, behavioral problems, being really sensitive to rejection, and severe issues with body image that go beyond what is normal for teenagers to feel.

It is discouraged to diagnose anyone who is younger than 18 with this disorder just because there are so many variables and mood changes in young adults and teenagers that it would be extremely easy to miss out or miss-diagnose someone who is just having their regular teenage concerns. This does not mean that the disorder cannot be diagnosed ahead of time, but it is usually dealt with in a case by case basis and most clinicians will not deal with at all until the person is 19. If it is diagnosed, the features will have to be present as well as consistent for a year or more before the diagnosis can be made.

If someone is diagnosed with this when they are a teenager, it is most likely going to predict that the person is going to have this same disorder when they are adults. Among those who were diagnosed with this disorder when they were younger, there is usually two groups; one is going to have the disorder and it is going to remain pretty stable over a period of time and then the other group that is going to have those who move in and also out of their diagnosis. An earlier diagnosis is sometimes helpful when trying to get an effective treatment plan in place, but since this kind of diagnosis is tricky, it is often not done. For those who are suffering from borderline personality disorder as teens, family therapy is usually the option that is the most preferred.

Diagnosing with Other Disorders

It is not uncommon for someone who is dealing with this kind of disorder to also have some other disorders, whether it is other personality disorders or something else, that are going to show up at the same time. This makes it even harder to find the personality disorder because it may be masked by some of the other symptoms that are there. Compared to those who have some of the other personality disorders, those who have borderline personality disorder are going to have a higher rate for also meeting the criteria for other disorders such as:

- Mood disorders—this is going to include things like bipolar disorder and major depression
- Anxiety disorders—there are a lot of these that can be met as well and would include post-traumatic stress disorder, social anxiety disorder, and panic disorder
- Other kinds of personality disorder
- Substance abuse

- Eating disorders—this would include things like bulimia and anorexia nervosa
- Attention deficit hyperactivity disorder
- Somatoform disorders
- Dissociative disorders

If a person with this personality disorder has one of these other issues, they should not be diagnosed with the personality disorder until that other issue has been dealt with. These other issues can give some of the same symptoms and sometimes taking care of these can be a simpler method of dealing with the personality disorder. This is unless the symptoms of the personality disorder can be proven to have been around for many years before the other issue came into play.

Also, it is more likely that women are going to experience some of the issues listed above while men will receive some of the others. For example, men are going to be higher with the substance use disorders while the women are going to have more of the eating disorders. It is important that you get these other disorders taken care of if you would like to see some of the best results with treating your borderline personality disorder. It is going to be pretty much impossible to take care of the personality disorder if you have some of the other issues listed above in the way because these are going to onset the disorder and will keep it going even with a lot of therapy in the process.

This is why most professionals will do a thorough examination of the patient to figure out if there are some other issues that are present in the patient. This can make it much easier to cure the personality disorder once the other issues are done. This can be done with some preliminary therapy or through the use of medications to treat issues such as like anxiety and depression for the best results.

Mood disorders

Many of those who suffer from this kind of disorder are also going to have some severe mood disorders. This is going to include things such as bipolar disorder and major depressive disorder. Some of the symptoms that come with borderline personality disorder are going to be similar to what you can find in mood disorders so this can make the diagnosis of the personality disorder difficult. It is very common for someone to get misdiagnosed; they will be told that they have bipolar disorder when they really have borderline personality disorder and it can go the other way as well.

For those who have bipolar disorder, they may have some of the symptoms of borderline personality disorder, but these symptoms are just going to appear while the person is going through one of their episodes and then they will go back to normal when the mood is stabilized. This is why it is so important that the clinician make sure that their client's mood is completely stable before they do their diagnosis.

For those who do not know much about either of the two disorders, they are going to look very much the same. Even some clinicians who study the two quite a bit are going to find that it is difficult, but there are a few differences that you can watch for that will help. First, the mood swings of the two are going to be different in their durations. For some people with bipolar, the episodes are going to last for a minimum of two weeks each time while the moods in someone with borderline personality disorder is going to last much less time. The mood switches in those with bipolar are going to take place over a series of days while the ones for BPD are going to change by the minute or hour.

Next, the moods that come with bipolar disorder are not going to be responding to changes that occur in the environment while the same is not true for borderline personality disorder. What this means is that for a person with bipolar disorder, their mood is not going to be lifted if there is a positive event in their lives while this kind of situation would have the potential to life the mood of someone with BPD. On the other hand, someone with bipolar disorder would not be brought down if they are really happy just because a bad event happens, but someone with BPD can easily be brought down at a moment's notice.

And then, when those with BPD are experiencing euphoria, they are going to do it without any racing thoughts and they are not going to have the need for less sleep. Often they are not going to have periods of sleep disturbance as well. On the other hand, those with bipolar are always going to have racing thoughts, trouble sleeping, and disturbances in their appetite.

This is why it is going to take some time for the clinician to determine if your loved one has a personality disorder or not. It is not as easy as it might look since there are some similarities in symptoms that the person is feeling and often they are just going to happen for different lengths or for different reasons. A thorough examination can help to determine if someone is suffering from true borderline personality disorder or if they are having issues with a mood disorder.

Premenstrual Dysphoric Disorder

Premenstrual Dysphoric Disorder, or PMDD, is a condition that can occur in some women and some of the symptoms are going to match up with what you can find in borderline personality disorder. It is estimated that between 3 and 8 percent of women are going to feel these symptoms and most of them are going to occur somewhere between 5 and 11 days before the period starts and then will go away after it has begun. There are quite a few symptoms that are similar to what you might find with borderline personality disorder and would include things like trouble with their relationships, difficulty with concentrating, binge eating, anxiety, and feeling like things are out of their control, feeling hopeless, depressed, irritability, and mood swings.

Most of the women who have PMDD will start to experience these kinds of symptoms when they are early on in their twenties, but it is often going to take them until they are in their thirties to get the treatment that they need. While some of the symptoms between BPD and PMDD are similar, they are two different things. They are going to be distinguished by the duration of the symptoms as well as the timing and the PMDD is not going to have issues with impulsivity.

Axis II Disorders

Over 66 percent of those who have borderline personality disorder are also going to have the right criteria for meeting another kind of personality disorder at some point during their lives. The most common would be the cluster a disorders like schizotypal, schizoid, and paranoid. The next common would be the cluster B disorders like narcissistic, histrionic, and antisocial disorders. In some cases they may have other issues such as obsessive compulsive disorder, dependent disorder, and avoidant disorder. These disorders could have occurred before the borderline personality disorder came about or they can show up afterwards during the treatment or a few years later.

The diagnosis of borderline personality can be difficult at times. If there are other underlying causes that are in the way, it can become difficult to determine what symptoms are from this personality disorder, and which come from the other issues that are present. Only a professional clinician will be able to determine if you or someone else has borderline personality disorder and the right steps that you will need to take in order to get the right treatment.

Chapter 5: Management and Prognosis

Once someone has been diagnosed with borderline personality disorder, it is time to learn how to manage the disorder. It is not going to go away just because it has been diagnosed and it can take years and years of proper therapy and treatment in order to get the condition under control and help the person suffering from the disease learn how to live a normal life. This chapter is going to take a bit of time to look at the different types of treatments that are available to choose from and how high the success rate is for the treatments.

Management

The main treatment that people with this disorder are going to receive is psychotherapy. Usually this will either be done on its own or with one of the other methods, but there are very few times when borderline personality disorder is treated without the use of psychotherapy. The treatment that is chosen though should be completely based on the individual needs of the person at hand rather than worrying about the traditional route that might have been taken by others. Sometimes medication will be the best option, for example, because it can help to treat some of the diseases that are going to come along with this disorder.

This section will look at some of the different types of treatments that are available for this kind of disorder, how each one of them is going to work, and when each of them is going to work for your situation.

Psychotherapy

The treatment that is used the most often with borderline personality disorder is psychotherapy. This is usually going to be done for long term. There are six different types of treatments that are currently recognized for this kind of therapy for the individual. They include schema-focused therapy, general psychiatric management, dialectical behavior therapy, or DBT, transference focused psychotherapy, metallization based treatment or MBT, and dynamic deconstructive psychotherapy or DDP.

The first type of therapy we will look at is the schema focused therapy. This is the type of therapy that is used the most often for this disorder, although the others can be used just as effectively. This is an approach that is going to add some of the best things about all of the other ones and tries to combine them. The schemas in this kind of therapy are going to be the themes or patterns of thinking, behaving, and feeling that the person has been using for a long time. These will be discovered in this kind of therapy and then the clinician will be able to work with the person in order to get them to change the way that they look at the world. These schemas will be formed from childhood and so they are deeply rooted and will take the person a lot of time in order to get them to change.

This kind of therapy is going to come in three stages. The first one is considered the assessment phase where the schemas are going to be identified over the first few sessions. These will often be determined through questions to the person in order to get a good picture of the patterns that are involved in their thoughts. Next the doctor is going to work with the patient in order to bring them to the emotional awareness that they need in order to understand and get in touch with the schemas and then they will learn the best way to spot them in their day to day life. Finally, the stage for behavioral changes will come about and the client is going to learn how to replace the negative thoughts of the past with ones that are new and healthy.

The next type of therapy is general psychiatric management. This is the kind of therapy that you could use on almost any kind of personality disorder that there is and it is going to work in order to help determine what kind of disorder is present and what the person is able to do in order to take care of the issue. It is a long process and it is not one that is specifically made for those who have borderline personality disorder, but it can do the trick and many times it is the only option for those who do not have access to a professional on their case.

Next therapy that is often used is dialectical behavior therapy. This is quickly becoming the most popular kind of therapy that is available because it is backed by a lot of research into borderline personality disorder and is going to help the client out the most. This is often considered the most effective treatment, but it is going to take a specialist who has been trained in using it and the client must be willing to stick with it for the long term. Often this is used in a kind of group therapy in order to make it more effective for those who need it.

The approach that is used with this is to change the behaviors and thoughts that have been around for many years with the patient. It is also a good one to use if the client is refusing to work with the therapist for the long term because it is able to put them at ease and make them feel less like they are under attack from the therapist. This kind of therapy will be given in two components, namely individual and group therapy. In the group part, the client is going to learn the skills that they need in order to make their life better. During the individual sessions, the therapist is going to work with them to identify and discuss any issues that the client might have dealt with in the past week. The therapist will record these and the help to devise a plan based on how the patient is concerned about it. The therapist will also spend some time talking about life skills and issues in these sessions. This along with some training to regulate emotions is used to put the client at ease and helps them to see that there are other alternatives to dealing with their problems.

Transference focused psychotherapy is sometimes used as well. This is kind of a general term for therapy, but it is basically when the client is going to talk out their issues, problems, and feeling with their therapist. During this kind of therapy, the client is going to learn about the condition that they are in as well as their behaviors, thoughts, feelings and moods. This kind of therapy is going to help them to learn the best ways to take control in life and teach them how to respond to any situations that are challenging with the right kind of coping skills rather than letting things get out of hand.

There are a variety of different types of this therapy and all of them are going to work in different ways. Some examples of this kind of therapy will include therapy, psychosocial therapy, counseling, and talk therapy. They are meant to get the client to talk out the issues that are surrounding them in order to make things easier to understand and change without the confrontations that can happen with other methods.

Next is the metallization based treatment. This therapy is a kind that is used to help the client separate and differentiate their thoughts and the feelings they are having from others around them. The metallization part is the ability to understand your own behavior and feelings as well as how you are associating them with your mental states in yourself and in others.

In this therapy, the client is going to learn how to do this process by using supportive and safe methods so that they do not feel like they are attacked. This process can take some time because the person with the disorder is going to become confused when things are changed on them and not going the way that they are used to. This one is going to take a specialist in order to get done and could take many years to accomplish.

Finally, some clinicians will use dynamic deconstructive psychotherapy to help out those with this kind of disorder. This is a treatment that can be used is usually only going to take about 12 months in order to complete with the client coming in every week to get the help that they need. This kind of therapy is going to combine a lot of different elements including the deconstruction philosophy, object relations theory, and neuroscience research. The ideas behind this type of therapy state that those who have this disorder need to work on the neurocognitive deficit so that they can start to properly process their feelings when things becomes emotionally charged.

For this therapy, the patient is going to show up for weekly sessions that will last about 45 minutes. Between the sessions, the client is going to be asked to work on some special assignments each day that the therapist asks them to fill out. They are also going to be asked to work on some of their own personal relationships when they are out of the treatment.

There are four stages and it is going to take 12 months. This does not mean that you will have a cured client in that 12 months, but it means that they are recovered enough to get out of such an intensive program and move on to more day to day living. If they are not to this point, the therapist will be able to block out more time to help them out.

No matter what kind of other treatment options that might be given to the patient, it is necessary for all patients to go through some form of therapy. Picking out the one that is right for the patient and is going to help them the most is the best option for everyone, but there should still be some kind of therapy present to get the best results. It is never recommended that the patient just be given medicine and then ignored because this is not going to give them the help that they need and they will never be cured.

Medications

In addition to working on therapy in order to help out with this disorder, some doctors may prescribe some medications to help out with the disorder. It is important to realize that medication on its own is not going to be able to help out the disorder and no one is going to get cured just by the medication that they have taken. Rather, the medication is usually used to help out with some of the underlying causes and issues that might be present so that it is easier to take care of the disorder and get the person back on the track that they belong.

There was a study done in 2010 that found that as of now there are no medications that are available for treating the core symptoms of borderline personality disorder. Even though this was found, the authors did find that some forms of medication are effective at helping the impact of some isolated symptoms or symptoms of the conditions that might be going along with the borderline personality disorder. What this means is that you are not going to be able to take a magic pill and get the results that you would like and be cured overnight, but some of the symptoms that you are feeling can be helped with medication which can make your treatment so much better in the long run.

There are some medications that you will be able to take in order to help with some of your symptoms. For example, haloperidol has been shown to reduce some of the anger that these clients may have and flupenthixol can reduce some of the likelihood that the client is going to have suicidal behavior. Aripiprazole can sometimes help out with the condition because it helps with anxiety, depression, paranoid symptoms, anger, impulsivity, and interpersonal problems. These are just some of the issues that medication can help with.

One of the things that medication is given out the most for when it comes to this personality disorder is the mood stabilizers. These can help out with anger, issues with relationships, anxiety, depression, and so much more. Often these are going to make it really difficult to take care of the person with the disorder and it becomes almost impossible to help them without the mood stabilizers.

Of course, the evidence that some of these medications have for helping out is a bit limited which is why some people who will not recommend these because they are worried about the safety of them. There are some guidelines in place in some countries concerning the management and treatment of this disorder. Basically, those who have the rules will say that the medications cannot be used as the sole treatment for someone who has this disorder and can only be used as part of the treatment to help along the more prominent option of therapy.

Medications are the best option if you need to deal with some of the underlying issues that are hindering the treatment of the disorder. They can take care of the other issues so that you are able to concentrate more on the treatment for your personality disorder. It is important that the medications are never taken on their own though and it is best to have them just as the supplement to the therapy in order to get the best treatment for all around. This will ensure that the patient is getting the best care, being monitored when needed, and that they can get off the medication as soon as it is no longer providing them with the benefits and care that it was meant for.

Services

While anyone who has this disorder is going to be able to benefit from treatment and getting the help that is available from a therapist or other doctor, most of those with this disorder are never going to get the help that they need. This is because most of them will not realize that they have an issue and the rest will not admit that they have an issue and will never seek the treatment that they need. Even for those who go and get the treatment that they need, it is hard to find a doctor who is going to be able to help them out the right way and they are not going to be able to get the good treatments that are available to some.

It is difficult for those who need to get the treatment to find the treatment options that they need. This is because of their location, the fact that they will need to be able to find the money to do treatments that they need and so they will take lower programs that will cost them less, and the fact that the services that they are going to receive will vary between the places that they get.

Managing the treatment of this disorder is going to be really tough. It is not something that can be done in just a short period of time and often it can take many years and a combination of different therapies and drugs in order to get it figured out. The client also needs to be willing to trust the clinician and stick with the treatment for a number of years, something that is difficult for someone with borderline personality disorder to properly do.

Prognosis

Out of those who get the treatment that they are needing when suffering from this disorder, the majority are going to do well and can get some relief from their symptoms and they will go into remission for at least two years if not longer. This is for those who went through the proper treatments and who stuck with it for the length of time that was required, something that is hard to get done for a person with borderline personality disorder.

According to a study that was done in order to track the symptoms of those who had this disorder and got the proper treatment, about 34 percent were in remission within two years of starting their treatment. After four years, this number went up to almost 50 percent and then within six years it was almost to 60 percent. By the end of this study, almost 74 percent of the participants were in remission. Out of those who had gotten to the recovery phase, less than 6 percent had gone backwards and began to see the same issues as they had before when they had the disorder. Another study that was done later found that after ten years of therapy and a change in lifestyle, a good 86 percent of the patients had gotten to a stable recovery from their symptoms.

What this shows you is that the majority of those who have undergone treatment are going to be able to see the results that they want as long as they are able to stick with the program and the amount of time that they have to spend in the program is going to vary depending on a variety of factors. Of course, there are some people who are not able to succeed in their goals and they are not going to be able to get through the therapy. Many times these people may not trust their therapist, may not see that there is a problem, or they were not able to stay for the length of the program in order to see the results of the participation.

These findings are contrary to what a lot of people have believed for many years. For a long time, people thought that it was impossible to get over borderline personality disorder, but with the right amount of treatment and time, it is possible to help reverse how these clients act in their world, even when they have some of the worst symptoms. These kinds of relief form the symptoms are only going to be possible for those who get treatment, regardless of the type and those who never receive treatment are not going to see the results that they would like.

The personality that the patient has is going to play a big role in how the therapy is going to go and if they are willing to trust the therapist and work with them for the long term, they are going to get much better outcomes in the process. some recent research shows that those with this disorder who have higher levels of agreeableness during therapies like dialectical behavior therapy, are more likely to get better outcomes compared to those who have a low agreeableness. This association is thought to be there because of the strength of the alliance that the therapist has made with the client. This means that the agreeable patients are able to develop the stronger alliances with the therapists which is needed in order to have better outcomes compared to those who were not considered as agreeable.

In addition to this, those who have this disorder are able to get better levels in terms of psychosocial functioning when they are given the treatment that they need to be better. A study that was done on this tracked the social as well as the work abilities of those who had this kind of personality disorder and found that after six years from being diagnosed, a good 56 percent of them were much better in their social and work environments. This is in comparison to the 26 participants who did well in social and work conditions before they got treatment right after diagnosis.

One thing to note is that vocational achievement is usually limited more, even compared to the other types of personality disorders that can be found. However, those who had symptoms that were remitted were much more likely to be in good relationships with their romantic partners and at least one of their parents, do better at school and work, were able to start working on their school and work history, and were much better with being in society.

As you can see, it looks pretty good for those who are getting the treatment that they need to deal with the symptoms of this personality disorder. But the important thing to realize is that they need to get the treatment to get help. Those with the disorder who do not get diagnosed or at least do not get the help that they need will never be able to see some of the results that are listed here. No one has been reported as being healed from this disorder working on their own, especially if they do not know they have the disorder, but the majority of those who have been treated are better and can become a better part of society.

While treatment is important, it is difficult to get for the person. They are not going to want to deal with the therapist or with admitting that they have something wrong. They may not want to deal with the long term relationship with the therapist and do not want to spend the next ten years in therapy. The important part is that those who love them the most and are always around need to show their support and love at all times to be the most helpful.

This is great news for everyone who is suffering from this disorder who wants to know that there is a light at the end of the tunnel. Everyone is going to go through a different amount of time that it will take to get through the treatment; some people are going to get done with it in just a few years while others can take the full ten years in order to see some results. The good news is that no matter how long it takes, it is more than likely if you stick with the program and do what you are supposed to, you will be able to see success. Even better, most of those who do see success are not going to have to worry about regression and going backwards. There is some hope as long as the patient is willing to keep going towards the final goal and getting the help that is needed.

Epidemiology

In the past, it was usually estimated that about 1 to 2 percent of the population would have this kind of disorder and that it would occur at least three time more for females than it would for men. It has been found that these numbers are quite a bit off. Of course, it is important to remember that these numbers are just guesses and are based off the number of people who have been diagnosed with the disorder; there are quite a few people who may have the disorder but who have never gotten the treatment that they need in order to get better.

Now it is estimated that out of the general population, 5.9 percent of them will have this kind of disorder and it will occur about 5.6 percent in men and 6.2 percent in women. The difference between men and female is so small that most researchers are not going to say that women are more likely to get it than men since the numbers are so high to start with.

In addition, this kind of disorder is often estimated to be the leading cause of at least 20 percent of hospitalizations that are considered psychiatric and it occurs in about 10 percent of the outpatients that are seen. In terms of how many inmates in prison have this disorder, it is estimated that 29.5 percent of the new inmates in the Iowa prison were fit into a diagnosis of the disorder in 2007 and it is estimated that the general population in US prisons would be around 17 percent. Perhaps if some of these people had been treated the way that they should have, they would have gotten the help that the needed and the prison system would be a whole lot emptier than it is now.

As you can see, there are a variety of different options when it comes to the treatment of this disorder and how much help that the person with the disorder is going to be able to get. It is pretty likely that if someone with this disorder reaches out and gets the help that is needed, they are going to be able to get a break from the symptoms that they are feeling and they can go on to live normal lives. They need to be willing to trust the therapist they are given though and to stick out what is all going to come. It is not an easy thing to do but with a bit of work and support, it is possible to give them the help that they need to live a good life.

Chapter 6: Steps to Take in Order to Deal with Borderline Personality Disorder

When you are dealing with borderline personality disorder, you need to make sure that you are getting the right steps down in order to get it taken care of and not allow it to take over your whole life. This is a serious condition that can affect a lot of your life but most people do not even realize that they are dealing with it. This could be due to the fact that they have been dealing with this condition for the majority of their lives and they just do not know any other way of thinking or feeling.

But getting diagnosed and getting the help that is needed is the most important step to take to get this under control and to have the ability to socialize properly with those around you. This chapter is going to look at some of the steps that you can take to help yourself with this disorder as well as some of the steps that family members can take if they start to see that something is wrong and they want to get their loved one some serious help.

What the Family Can Do

There are some things that the family is going to be able to do in order to take care of the issue and to show that they are there for the one whom they love. This is a trying time for the family as well as the person who is going through this disorder and this is not something that should be ignored for either of them. Often the family is going to become angry at the person who is going through the disorder and so they are not going to be able to show the sympathy that is needed for the person nor the support. But often the strain that is put on the family is great too and this should be taken care of along with the issues that the person with the disorder is going through.

There are a number of steps that can be taken in order to help out the person who has this disorder. The family is going to be the best help possible if they are willing to still hold onto their love for them and not blame the person rather than the disorder for the issues. The following are some of the steps that you can take to help out with this issue.

Recognize the Problem

The first thing that you will need to do is recognize that there is a problem. While this might seem like it is something that is really easy to do and should not take a lot of time and effort, it is actually one of the hardest things to do. There are usually two reasons why the family members might not recognize that there is an issue going on with their loved one; they may be in denial that something is present or they may not be around the person enough, since the person shoved them away, to notice that something is wrong.

Let's look at the first issue. The family members may be in a bit of denial about the fact that their loved one is going through the issue. They may think that it is just a phase or they are scared to admit that something is wrong with someone in their family. There can also be the issue that once they know about the problem, they are scared that by mentioning it, they are going to lose all contact with the person they love and this can scare them in return. But it is important to recognize the signs as soon as possible and then to realize that the person is going to need your help. Do not blame them for the way that they may have treated you in the past and instead spend some time realizing that they have a big issue and need some help. Think of it this way, you would not blame someone for getting cancer and make them feel bad about it so why would you blame someone who has borderline personality disorder.

The second issue is that the family members may not be close enough to the sufferer any more in order to see that something is going on. They may have noticed something was funny at one point but then they might not at all. Sometimes they will find that they said something to the sufferer just once and then they were not talking anymore and the family member is left confused and dazed.

When you have nothing to do with the sufferer, it is really hard to tell that something is going wrong and often the issue is not going to be resolved. If something like the situation described above happens, it is a good idea to check with other family members and perhaps some friends of the sufferer to see if they have had contact with the sufferer recently. Most of those with this kind of disorder are going to have a lot of issues with keeping relationships of any kind so it is often a good indicator of a problem if you are not able to find any of their old friends are still talking to them.

If any of this begins to happen to you, it is best to get them the help that you can as soon as possible. This is going to take some work, but if you and a few family members get together and work it out a bit, you may be able to convince them to give it a try rather than to just take their anger out on you for the suggestion. Recognizing the problem is the first step that you can take in order to help out your loved one as soon as possible.

Be Understanding

You also need to be understanding of the person who has this disorder. They are not able to control the feelings that they are having and since most of it is in their brains, from genetics, a part of their past, and just something that they have had to deal with for the majority of their lives, they really do not see that the things they are doing are wrong since they are used to them completely. You need to understand that this is not something that they are just able to turn off and on and it is going to take a lot of time and understanding before they are able to change the way that they are thinking.

There are a lot of times when the family of the sufferer are going to be upset when they are dealing with the sufferer, but they get even angrier when they find out the actual condition that is causing the issue. While this might seem like something that does not make much sense, it could be due to the fact that they are given the wrong information about the disorder and so they are not able to understand what it is all about.

If you have someone you know who is dealing with this disorder, it is important that you get all of the information that you can about it in order to help out your loved one. This guidebook is a good place to start and it is able to make you understand a bit more about this disorder so that you can help out your loved one much more efficiently. This is going to be a long road for the both of you, but with a bit of hard work and understanding between the both of you, the easier it is going to be to get through it.

The best thing that you are going to be able to do for your loved one is just to understand what they are going through. This is not something that they are doing on purpose and in most cases, they are not even going to realize that they are doing it or causing harm to others. It is not something that they did to themselves and without therapy, it is not something that they can get rid of. Your understanding is a great way to encourage them to get the help that is needed to see some great results.

Do Not Blame the Person, Blame the Disorder

It is easy for some of the family members to start blaming the person who has the disorder rather than blaming the disorder that is causing all of the trouble. They may think that this is something that the person should have been able to deal with or stop on their own and they do not understand all that is going on with this person. They are going to hold the person with the disorder to blame for the mistakes and the issues that are present and this is not going to help anyone.

Placing the blame in the wrong place is the worst thing that you can do in this situation. You need to take the time to realize that this is not the fault of your loved one but rather it is the fault of the disorder that they are dealing with. While this may be something that is hard to understand, you will be able to get through it together much better if the disorder can be your common enemy. Do not turn away your loved one because you think that they are the ones to blame for this whole thing. They do not have much of a say in what is going on and often they are just as lost and confused as you are in the whole thing. Blame the disorder and things become a lot easier to handle and understand and the two of you can begin to work together to make it right.

Seek Treatment and Help for Your Loved One

Once the disorder has been found out, it is time to get your loved one the treatment that they need. This needs to be done as soon as possible. Your loved one is never going to get better if they never get any treatment and in most cases they are going to get worse. While treatment does take a long time to get through, it is much better to get through this because most cases are going to see a full recovery over some time. This is great news if you are looking to see if there is a light at the end of this very long tunnel.

Before sending them in to get some help, make sure that you are doing your research. You want to find someone who is going to understand what your loved one is going through and you will want to make sure that they are at least a little bit trained in dealing with this issue. A lot of the reason that some people fail is because their therapist just did not have the right training or knowledge in order to help them out. Try to find someone who knows what they are doing and you will see that this is much easier to handle for the both of you.

One thing to keep in mind though, you need to remember that your loved one is going to be a little bit resistant to the idea of therapy. They do not think that they have any problems and so they are going to shy away from getting this help. They might be worried that having this disorder is going to make them less of a person or that others are not going to like them as much. But you need to find a way to make them understand that this is the best for them and that this is going to make their lives so much better. It is not going to be an easy road, but with a good therapist, especially one that your loved one can trust, you will find that it is much easier and more successful and your loved one is going to be on the right path to success in no time at all.

Seek Treatment and Help for You and Other Loved Ones

Not only is your loved one going to need to get some support and therapy, but you and others who have been close to the person with the disorder will need to go and get the support that is needed. Most families assume that they just need to get support for the loved one and then everything will be fine, but this is not always the case. You have probably been through a lot with this journey; many people who go through borderline personality disorder will be mean and violent against their loved ones and act out at just the slightest issue imaginable. This can be hard on the family, most of whom do not understand what is going on and are feeling lost and hurt because of the situation.

When you have gone through all of this with your loved one, it is important to realize that you have been hurt and that you do deserve to have someone on your side. For those who feel like they have been betrayed by their loved one and that they would benefit from it, there are a lot of options for therapy that are going to make it easier to understand what all is going on and some can even teach you the proper way to help yourself as well as the one that you love.

Make sure that you pick out the therapy that makes you the most comfortable. There are a lot of different options that are out there and none of them are necessarily right or wrong, but it is more a matter of personal taste and what you would like to see. Some people like to have the one on one attention that comes from individual therapy and others like to work with a group to get their feelings out. It does not matter which therapy you choose, just make sure that you are also getting the help that you need to feel better about the whole situation and to start to realize what is going on.

Be Supportive Through the Journey

The most important thing that you can do for your loved one is to be as supportive as possible through this journey. This is not an easy time for them. They are being told that the way that they act and think is not normal and that they need to get it taken care of, and they are probably very confused. This is the only way that they have been for a long time and it is scary to think that you are doing something that is wrong and that you have a personality disorder. Think of how badly you would feel if you were told you had this kind of disorder. You probably would not feel all that good and neither does your loved one.

So while you are going through this journey with your loved one, take a step back and realize that this is not the easiest thing in the world for them as well. You may think that they are just acting out and causing problems, but in reality they are just confused and do not know what to do. But if they see that you are going to be there to help them out all of the time and that you are on their side, they are going to feel so much better about themselves and their lives. Your support is a big determining factor in whether they will get and stay with the treatment they are getting and if they are going to be successful in their recovery.

These are just a few of the steps that you can do in order to help your loved one with this disorder realize what is going on and to get them the help that they really need. This is not an easy process for anyone who is involved so take the process slowly and understand that it is going to take some time and some healing before everything is better.

What the Person with Borderline Personality Can Do

As the person who is going through this situation, you are the one who will be affected the most by what is going on. It can be difficult to know what to do when everyone around you is saying that the way you act, think, and behave are not normal and that you have something that is a personality disorder. To the ones who have this disorder, these characteristics are not out of the normal. Their brains have bene wired in a way that this all seems to be normal. As seen with some of the causes that are listed above, the brain may have the sufferer acting like this just because they are trying to protect them from things that occurred in the past or they may just have hormones that are sending the wrong message and so they think this is all normal.

It can also be hard to deal with the fact that all of the things you have had to deal with for your entire life have been wrong. These people might feel like they are putting all of the blame on you, out to get you, or just do not understand. But letting them in and following the steps that are listed below will help you to get the treatment and help that you need so that you can go back to a natural and healthy life that includes more relationships and steady emotions.

Be Aware of the Issue

The first thing that you will need to do in order to get this personality disorder taken care of is to be aware that there is an issue at hand. This is going to be the hardest part, but if you are not willing to get the help that is needed, you are never going to get through this issue no matter how much someone else may want you to.

Since you are used to the way that you think and it is the way that you have done things for years, it is going to be hard to let it all change. You are used to thinking this certain way and these tendencies have been rooted in you perhaps since you were a young child. Often these thoughts will be this way because your brain is trying to protect you from something that has happened in the past or something that it wants to protect you from now, so you are not getting in all of the information that you need; this results in you making poor decisions because you just do not have all of the information.

If someone is trying to help you out, you should try to figure out if they are right. You will have to take the time to figure out how they are related to you and if they have your best interests at heart. If they are a close family member who has been around you for years but you have spurned off for some reason or another in recent times and yet they are still concerned for you, it might be time to sit down and see if they are telling something that is the truth. At least be open to learning more about the condition and perhaps having a few conversations with a specialist to see if this might be something that could be related to you.

Understand others are trying to Help

Sometimes it may feel like the others who are around you are just there to attack the way that you think and do things. It may not feel like they have the right frame of mind when they are talking to you or that they understand all of the hard things that you are going through. This is natural to feel this way. You are used to seeing people in certain ways and sometimes people who you cut out of your life a long time ago are going to start coming back and acting like they are trying to help you. This can be confusing and is going to put you on your guard. Plus, who wants to be told that they have a personality disorder and need to get some professional help to get better?

Try not to get offended when someone tries to help you out with this problem, even if you do not think that it is something of their concern or that you have this disorder. Try to look at it from their perspective. They think that they are helping you out with this information and they have let down their guard, especially if the two of you have not been speaking for some time, and they are trying to get you the help that you need. They are not trying to track or trick you in this process, they just want to be on your side and help you out.

Be Open to Treatment

To be able to feel better and get back the normalcy that is going to make your life much better and open up so many more doors than before, it is important that you learn how to be open to treatment. This might be something that is scary for you, or you might think that it is not worth your time because you do not think that you have an issue to deal with in the first place. But sometimes it is hardest to see that there is a problem when you are so close to the action and so give it a try. If someone is so worried about you that they think you need help from a specialist, it is best to give it a try and see what it is all about.

Going to a few sessions is just going to take up a bit of your time and there are a wide variety of counseling types that you can choose for. Be open to the idea of treatment and perhaps try out a sessions of the one that sounds the most interesting to you. Of course, you may be stuck with just one or two options depending on the area where you live and the options that they have, but you are going to get the chance to talk about some of your feelings, about your life, and see if this is an issue that you are going to have to take care of.

Do not worry, if you do not have this disorder, you are going to be out of the clinician's office in no time. They have a few tests, as well as taking some time to talk to you, that are going to help to determine pretty quickly if you have this kind of disorder. If not, they will send you home and there is no issue. But if you do have this disorder, they are going to be able to tell it as well as the extent that you are dealing with it and they can give you some of the help that you need.

Take the first couple of sessions that you are doing with the clinician to find out if you will be comfortable with them and how you are both going to be able to work together. Do you feel comfortable and do you think that you will like the style that they are presenting when you work towards treatment? If something just does not go well for you, other than the fact that you do not want to be there, then request that you go with someone else. You have to be willing to put in a bit of the work in the process if you would like to see some of the great results.

Do not be scared about whether the treatment is going to work or not. This is one of the things that scares those with this disorder the most. They worry that they are going to put in a lot of effort to cure a disorder that they did not even know they had just to find out that they are not going to succeed in the long run. Going in with this kind of mind frame is going to make your success harder to get. Just go in with an open mind and listen to what the clinician is trying to do with you. This is going to help you get the treatment that you need the most efficiently. Most of those who work with the clinician and try to get better are going to see the success that they are looking for.

Trust and Worth with Your Therapist

If you want to have any chances of this kind of treatment and therapy to work at all, you need to learn how to trust your therapist. This is harder than it might seem at first because many people have issues with trusting anyone. When it comes to their therapist, this issue may get worse because they feel that the therapist is against them or that they are being judged for no reason.

Keep in mind that the therapist is there to work with you. Some people with borderline personality disorder are going to start out on a good foot with their therapist and then a few months down the line will either quit wanting to work at all with them in the sessions or they might not show up anymore. This could have been from some little thing that the therapist said that would have upset the client.

As the client, you need to remember that things are not always black and white like you would like them to be and that the therapist is really on your side even if there are times when they say things that you are not that fond of. Before you even get started on doing therapy with them, you need to go to a few sessions and see how the two of you get along. While a particular therapist may be one of the best in the area, if you are not going to get along with them or trust them, they are not going to be able to help you out at all. Take the first few sessions to find someone who is able to work well with you and who is going to be able to get you through the long road to recovery.

Follow the Assignments that are given

While you are in your sessions, you are going to be spending a lot of time with your therapist talking about your feelings and the way that you see things as well as learning a few new tactics for changing the way that these things work. There might also be some talk to determine if you have other disorders that might be in the way, or at least making the issue worse, when it comes to your personality disorder. There are going to be a lot of things packed into each of your sessions and sometimes it can seem overwhelming, but you will get used to it.

Outside of your sessions, there is going to be some work that you will have to do as well. Your therapist is going to give some kinds of assignments that they would like you to work on in order to help with the process. It is never a good idea, especially when you are right in the beginning of your sessions, to spend just one hour a week with the therapist and then go back to your normal way of life once the session is over. This is not going to help you out for very long and it is most likely that you are going to revert back to some of the old habits that you had until you get back to the therapy session the next week.

This is why your therapist is often going to hand out things of homework in order to do in between the sessions. These assignments are going to be useful because they are going to build upon the things that you were working on in the sessions so that they stay fresh in your mind and you are actually getting some experience with seeing them work in real life. You need to have these new lessons presented to you each day for the long term if you would like to see the results and even if it would be nice to get it just for an hour once a week, this is not going to give you the results that you are looking for.

When your therapist gives you an assignment at the end of your session, make sure that you take it seriously and try to work on it a bit each day. Yes this is going to feel like you are back in school again, but in the long run it is all going to be worth it. The harder that you are willing to do the work during the process the quicker and more likely your success is going to be and soon you will be on the right road to seeing your new life.

Stay for the Long Term for Best Results

The road to your recovery is not going to be easy and it is not going to be done in the amount of time that you would like. This is a long road that will take a lot of time and for most people it is going to take at least a few years though it could take up to 10 years depending on the age of the client and how bad their borderline personality disorder is when they finally go in to get the help they need.

While this might seem like a long time, you have to remember that this is a process that is trying to change the way that your brain thinks and acts. This took a long time to get started in the brain and so it is going to take a bit of time in order to get your brain back to the right place where it belongs. Many of the clients that go through therapy are not ready for the amount of time and effort that they have to put into all of this and so they may get frustrated. They might think that they will only need to take a few sessions in order to get all fixed and ready to go. For the most part, those who fail with their therapy are the ones who either did not trust their therapist to start with or they are the ones who were not ready for the time commitment and who got frustrated before leaving.

If you would like to see the great results that have been promised to those who have been working towards their success, you need to be there for the long term. There is no skipping out early, partial recovery, or anything else like that. You either need to stay in it for the whole time, no matter how long it might take, or you will not see the success that you were hoping to find when coming to therapy. It is that simple.

Begin to Live Your New Life

After you have done all of the steps that are listed above, it is time to take a step back and begin to live the new life that you have been given. This is going to be a bit tough for some people but the road to recovery is going to be a great one if you put in all of the effort that was required to get there.

Sometimes it will take quite a while to realize how far you were able to get through this process. It was not a process that took just a few months and you can go back on and see that things have changed. This is a process that most likely took quite a few years and it is hard to look back on all of the things that have changed in order to compare. But if you did all of the therapy that you were required to have and worked hard on fixing your life, there is going to be a change in you that others will see as well.

First, you are going to have a better time with the relationships that are in your life. You may have already made up with some of the family and friends who you had gotten rid of years before through your therapy. You are also going to notice that the next romantic relationship that you get into is going to work out so much better than you have ever found in the past. This can give your life so much more in terms of fulfillment and happiness that you would not have expected in the past and a lot of the feelings of abandonment will be gone from your life when it was there before.

Next, your thoughts of being worthless and thinking about self-harm will be pretty much gone. You are going to start feeling like you are worth something, you will be better at the job that you are doing or at school, and you are going to have friends and family who get along with you again so your outlook on life is going to be a lot better than before. When you stick with the therapy and do the work that is asked of you, it is going to become a lot easier to get these things for your own life.

When you are done with therapy, you are going to see that things are not always in black and white. You will understand that people have things that are going on in their lives and they are not ignoring you just because they need to go do something else at that moment. You will start to see that things are not always the way that you used to see them and that everyone has their own point of view. This new way of thinking is going to make it easier to keep your opinions in check and live a happier life.

Finally, you are going to find out that your emotions are going to be much more in check when you are done with your therapy. This is going to be something that is really new to you. Instead of going up and down over every little thing, you will find that instead you can just stay in one place and feel happy when things are good and not as sad when things are not going the way that you would like. You can also feel happier more often which is going to be a nice change from the emotions that you may have had in the past.

The emotions will not be as intense which can give you a much better outlook on your life and will show that the therapy was really worth all of that time.

As you can see, there are a few steps that both the family members and the sufferer of this disorder are going to be able to do in order to try and make things better. Often figuring out that there is an issue is the first thing that is going to have to happen. When that is done, it is going to take a lot of support and working together in order to help out everyone who is involved. It is a lengthy process that will take some work, but the outcomes will bring everyone close together and make them much better for it.

Chapter 7: Controversies with Borderline Personality Disorder

There are a lot of different controversies that can surround this kind of personality disorder. Many people feel like there is a kind of stigma around it that makes it really hard to get the person they help that they need. They have heard about this stigma in some sort or another so they are not willing to get the help that they need since they are not going to admit that there is an issue. Others are not going to be willing to help because they think that the sufferer is just full of themselves and should be able to get the help that is needed just from changing their own thoughts.

While it is not that easy, there are a lot of controversies that can come with this kind of personality disorder. These talk about whether the person with this kind of disorder is actually going to be able to get help or will they lie to get through it as well as some of the different ways that this and other personality disorders are portrayed in the media and popular literature. It is meant to give a few other points of views when it comes to this kind of disorder and also shows why it is so hard for some people to get the help that they need.

Credibility in Terms of Testimony from Those with Borderline Personality Disorder

Whether you are able to believe a person who has this kind of disorder has been something that people have been questioning for years. There are two concerns that people have with this kind of things and these include that a key condition of the condition is lying and that there are many dissociative episodes that they can face as well, both of which are going to make it difficult for them to get the treatment and help that they need in order to start feeling a bit better. This section will explore each of these in a bit more details to help with determining if they are valid concerns or not.

Dissociation

It is uncertain whether the process of dissociation is a part of this personality disorder and if it is used to impact the ability of the sufferer of borderline personality disorder to remember past events or the specifics of these events when needed. Even those who have researched this for years have trouble figuring out what is going on. Dissociation, to help it make a bit more sense, is a feeling of being detached from the physical experiences or emotions.

There was a study done during 1999 that showed haw the specificity of the autobiographical memory appeared to be decreased in those with this kind of personality disorder. The researchers of this same study also found that the amount of specifics that the person could recall would be correlated with how dissociated the person was at the time.

While this might seem like it is a bit hard to understand. In this disorder, there are times when the person is going to become detached from the things that are going on around them. This is something that will happen to others at times, but usually only when they are feeling harmed or going through something that is really hard to deal with. They are attached from the experience so that they will be able to get through it a bit better than they would if they have to live it. This can make it difficult to remember what exactly was going on in this period.

For the person with borderline personality disorder, this is going to work a bit differently. They are going to go into this kind of state easier because they will get worried about something or something is going to make the brain think that they are going to be harmed. While in this state, they will have some troubles with remembering the specifics of what is going on right now as well as the things that were going on in the past.

When someone is not able to remember the facts about their lives, even if it is just for a short amount of time, how are they going to get the help that they need in order to get better? This is one of the controversies that is around the treatment of this kind of disorder. It is almost impossible to know all of the time when someone is going through this dissociation and so the clinician could be working with them while the sufferer, who may feel like they are under attack, is not going to be answering in the way that is the most truthful or honest because they are blocking out their feelings.

This is an issue that is furthered complicated by the fact that even the researchers and those who are close to the cause are not able to figure out. Some think that this is a big deal and want to find a way to work around it while others do not think it has much if any impact and want to continue to treat their patients the way that they have been doing so far.

Lying as a feature

The basis for this one is how you can help someone who is always lying to you and never telling the truth. The matter gets more complicated when the person is only lying to you some of the time instead of all of the time because you have to figure out when they are saying something that makes sense or when they are just making things up to give you what you would like to hear rather than what is really going on.

There are some theorists in the field who believe that those who have this kind of disorder are the ones who are going to lie the most often. They think that the client is going to say the things that their doctor wants to hear so that they are able to get off the hook and get back to the things they were doing in the past. They will say what is wanted rather than worrying about getting the help that they need.

There are others who have worked with their patients for a long time who say that they rarely if ever see their patients with borderline personality disorder lie when it comes to the clinical practice. Regardless of which one might be right, the act of lying is not recognized as a criteria for this disorder so it is not as likely to have an effect on what is going on in the sessions together.

The biggest issue with the idea that those with this disorder are always lying is that it could affect the amount and type of care that the person is going to be receiving. Many times if it is believed that the person is lying during their sessions, they are not going to get as good of healthcare or they may be ignored when it comes to their health or their legal matters. This can put them in a dangerous predicament because no one is going to want to help them and they will really need that help.

Let's take a look at an example of this. The story of Jean Goodwin is a good option to use. This is a patient who was diagnosed with multiple personality disorder, or as it is now known as dissociative identity disorder. This patient suffered from some pain in her pelvic area because of some traumatic events that occurred when she was a child. Rather than believe the things that she was telling them, the doctor's thought that she was lying and diagnosed the issues as borderline personality disorder because they thought that lying was one of the key features you would find in this disorder.

Because of this kind of diagnosis that included frequent lying, even though the diagnosis was wrong, there were later issues that came up. At one point the patient had told doctors that she was allergic to the adhesive tape they were going to use during her surgery. The doctors did not believe her and thought that she was overdramatic due to the kind of diagnosis that she was given and so they used the adhesive tape. The patient had not been lying and there ended up being some complications during the surgery because the doctors had used it.

The biggest issue here is the thoughts that go behind diagnosing someone with borderline personality disorder. This shows that even those who work the closest with those who have the disorder have the wrong kinds of thoughts with it so why should the general public have any different thoughts. It is important to realize that lying is not one of the traits that is found with this disorder; while they may say some things that are not the most true, such as their mother hates them when really she was just trying to get them the help at the clinic, this is more because their brain sees things in a different way rather than they are trying to trick you or because they do not want to get in trouble.

Since lying is not considered one of the issues that comes with this disorder, it needs to be treated in a different way than you would for someone who was a chronic liar. This is going to ensure that the person with borderline personality disorder is getting the help that they need instead of being miss-diagnosed.

Gender

Even gender is under fire for determine who has this disorder and who does not. Even among those in the health care industry it is believed that more women are going to suffer from the disorder than men. While the percentage points for women are slightly higher, it is really not enough to make a difference and for the most part it is almost even between whether men or women will get this disorder.

The first thing to remember is that even in the mental health community, there is a big stigma about this kind of disorder. Sometimes it is so bad that some of those who were diagnosed with borderline personality disorder and were also childhood sexual abuse survivors can end up traumatized all over again just because of the negative ways they are treated by their health care provider. This is regardless of the gender who is being presented for the case.

There are two camps that are used to help determine why more women than men are diagnosed with this personality disorder and this is often more of the fact that women might be diagnosed with this disorder when they have the symptoms while men with the same symptoms might be diagnosed with other disorders such as post-traumatic stress disorder. One of the camps says that it is much better to give a diagnosis, whether it is for men or for women, of PTSD. This diagnosis is better in some cases because it can be used to acknowledge that there is some abuse that is controlling the behavior of the sufferer. Those who are against this kind of diagnosis argues that it is going to make abuse a medical issue rather than letting it address the causes in society that could be making this condition worse for the sufferer.

Regardless of which camp of though you are in, using PTSD as a diagnosis is not going to take into consideration of all the symptoms that come with the disorder so it is not really a good option to use in order to try and get this all taken care of. Despite this, some doctors and clinicians are still diagnosing it as PTSD and this diagnosis could affect how many women have personality disorders compared to men.

In some estimates, it is believed that out of the people who are diagnosed in the clinic with borderline personality disorder, 80 percent of them are women. Of course, it is recognized that the number is not going to be this high outside of the clinic and in most estimations the amount of women and men with the disorder are going to end up being pretty even rather than this spread out.

So why are there such big differences between the women who are diagnosed with this disorder and the men? It is believed that it is because the women are the ones who are coming in when they have the symptoms. Women are much more likely to show the symptoms of borderline personality disorder that are going to bring them in for some treatment. For example, depression is one of the signs and twice as many women are going to have this disorder compared to the men. Many women with depression will get help or someone is going to bring them in to get the help that they need, giving the doctor the time to examine them and perhaps make the BPD diagnosis.

This does not mean that men are not showing symptoms, they are just showing some of the other symptoms and these are not ones that most people will go to the doctor for. For example, men who have this disorder are more likely to show issues of psychopathy and substance abuse. They may not go in so the doctor is not able to check them out and see if there is actually a problem that is present.

Also, the way that men and women show their distress is going to come out in different ways. Men are more likely to drink in excess and they will carry out a larger amount of crimes. On the other hand, women will turn the anger inside to themselves which is going to lead them to depression and the act of self-harm that is found in some patients with this disorder. The men are probably going to be more likely to end up in jail for the things they are doing with this disorder while the women, or at least their friends force them, go into the doctor and seek the help that is needed.

In addition, it seems that men are not as likely to seek the help that is needed. There was a study done in 1994 that showed that between the ages of 18 to 35, 30 percent of the suicides that happened were with those who had borderline personality disorder. The fact that they had this disorder was confirmed through an autopsy and the symptoms were discussed with various family members. Most of those in the 30 percent were men and most of those were not in treatments. The amount of women in the group was much smaller.

So in conclusion, the men are not as likely as the women to seek or get the appropriate treatment that they need. This means that the numbers for them are done because they are never going in to get the diagnosis that they need. In addition, they have different symptoms of this disorder, such as substance abuse, and sometimes they are going to cause severe self-harm before they are able to get help.

Women on the other hand are going to get more of the help that they need because their symptoms are easier to recognize amongst their friends and family and this is the main reason why their numbers are so much higher. The amount of people of both genders who have the disorder is probably pretty similar, but the fact that they are not being diagnosed and that their symptoms are different from what is expected, it is less likely that the men are getting the help they need.

Manipulative Behavior

The kind of behavior that is used to determine if someone has borderline personality disorder is sometimes under scrutiny. There are a lot of people who think that those with borderline personality disorder will use manipulative behavior in order to influence things to be the way that they want. But this is also leading to the assumption that those with this disorder are causing themselves harm and thinking about suicide just so they can get people to do something that they want.

This is still under a lot of scrutiny because it is sometimes not believed because most of the time, those with borderline personality disorder are not able to control the emotions that they have, much less try to control the emotions that others have. This chapter is going to look at the facts about manipulative behavior and if it is really something that is found in this disorder and should be used in order to treat it.

The use of manipulative behavior in order to get the nurturance that the person needs is considered one of the characteristics of those who have borderline personality disorder by many of those who are in the mental health profession. However, as mentioned before, this is insinuating that those with this kind of disorder and who are communicating their intense pain, engaging in self-harm, and going through suicidal behavior, are doing this because they are in the process of influencing others. The impact of the behaviors of the therapist, family members, and friends is often assumed to be the intentions from the beginning and can change the way that the therapist and others are looking at and treating them.

Despite the prevalent thought among those in the field, those who have this disorder often do not have the ability that is necessary to manage their interpersonal challenges and painful emotions. The fact that they show intense pain, suicidal behavior, and self-harm is more about trying to regulate their moods or to get out of a situation that they cannot bear rather than trying to cause harm or manipulate someone else. They are left with nowhere else to turn and often the way that others see them during this process is the furthest thing from their minds.

For example, you can look at this in two ways. The first, you are going to see someone who is hurting themselves and threatening to do things if someone they love does not comply in some way. You are going to see this person as someone who is manipulative and who is going to do anything that they can in order to get the final outcome that they are looking for. On the other hand, if you see someone who is hurting themselves because they are upset and sad and do not know what else to do, you may feel a bit more compassion for them and want to give them the best treatment possible.

This is kind of where it is left off with the mental health professional. If they see the person with this personality disorder as manipulative and out to get them, they are going to offer a different form of therapy and they might always be on the guard against what is coming their way. If they see the person as someone who just needs help getting away from the emotions, they might feel a bit more empathy during the sessions and they are more likely to try and help you in a more kind fashion that could help.

The controversies that come up from this is that the way a doctor perceives the issue is going to change the way that they treat the patient. There needs to be a better understanding of what is going on with this kind of disorder. If the patient is being treated like they are an evil person who is out to get the therapist, it is not likely that they will trust the therapist and the treatment is never going to be successful.

Stigma

The stigmas that come with this kind of personality disorder are going to make it hard to give the sufferer the kind of treatment that they need. Some of the features of this disorder, including the fear of being rejected, the intense need to be intimate with those around them, unstable relationships with others around them, and the emotional instability, can often make others around the sufferer feel intense emotions as well. There are a lot of terms that are used around those with this personality disorder, that are going to make their treatment more difficult because they invoke certain responses in others. Some terms used include attention seeking, demanding, manipulative, and treatment resistant.

No matter how good you are at your job of doing health care, if you heard some of the terms above to describe a patient you were going to deal with, you probably would not be that excited. These terms are going to become self-fulfilling because the sufferer is not going to get the treatment that they need and then they are going to trigger more behaviors that are destructive to themselves.

Below are some examples of the more prevalent stigmas that are found for those with this kind of personality disorder and why they can be controversial when it comes to getting the person the treatment they need.

Physical Violence

There is a lot of stigma that is with this disorder when it comes to the idea of physical violence. Most of those who have never dealt with someone who has this disorder will assume that the sufferer is going to be really violent not only to themselves but also to the others who are around them. This is not because of what they know about the disorder but more because they will see this kind of behavior portrayed in various visual media and in the movies. Despite the popular belief and stigma, most of the researchers will agree that those with this disorder are not very likely to cause harm to others.

Yes, it is true that those with borderline personality disorder are going to have a lot of trouble dealing with their emotions and they are going to show intense anger at times, they are going to be more likely to direct it to themselves rather than to someone else. This means that they are going to cause themselves harm or think about suicide before they would even think of causing harm to someone else.

One of the reasons that people with this disorder are not going to consider hurting other people is because they were abused in their childhood. This will result in them adopting a no tolerance idea when it comes to expressing their anger to others in any method. They are averse to violence because of the way that they were treated when they were younger and so they will not be able to cause harm, express their needs well, or show any kind of assertiveness. Any anger that they do show is going to be shown to themselves and the others around them are never going to be harmed physically.

Notice the use of physical violence above. Some of the family members of those who have this disorder can be hurt in an emotional way though. They are going to see their loved ones hurting or they may be abandoned by their loved ones and not know what is going on. This can cause some hurt, but it is going to be in the form of the emotions and not with any physical harm since those with borderline personality disorder are not often, if ever, going to show any of this kind of violence to others.

Mental Healthcare Professionals

Those who have this kind of disorder are often considered some of the hardest patients to work with when it comes to therapy. It is thought that they are going to need a lot of skill as well as training for the therapists and others who are involved in helping them out. This is another of the stigmas that are around those with this kind of personality disorder and it is one that can be true in some cases. A majority of the therapists and others who work with those with this kind of disorder will say that these clients are sometimes difficult and are amongst the hardest out of all the other groups they work with. Perhaps this is because of the attitude to those who have this disorder or it may be because they are hard to deal.

In some theories, it is believed that the person with this kind of personality disorder is so hard to deal with because of the ideas that the therapists and others who work with the sufferer hold when they walk in the door. They think that the client is going to be difficult and so the client becomes difficult whether that is actually the case or not. Think of it this way, have you ever dreaded going to some place or doing something. It is not likely that you enjoyed yourself all that much because of the notions you already had in place but if you had been a little more upbeat and open, it might have gone a little better.

This is why it is often believed that the negative experience that is happening in the sessions is more the fault of the outlook the clinician already has than it is about how the client is acting.

Why is this such a bad thing? Because it can end up with the wrong course of treatment for the patient which can lower their chances of being able to get better. The doctor is seeing behavior that is not there, or at least not as bad as they think it is, and so they are giving the wrong sorts of treatment such as punitive interpretation and limit setting, inappropriate mothering, and using too much medication for a problem that may not need medication to start with. This is making it more difficult for the client to get better and it is going to result in both the client and the doctor giving up on the treatment before it is even done.

Terminology

Sometimes the terminology that comes with this kind of disorder can be the biggest issue that is at hand. Often the issues that are above are going to make it a discussion on whether the term of borderline personality disorder should be renamed into something that is friendlier and does not cause the same kind of issues as what the current name does. Some feel that the current name is just fine and does not cause the issues that are being discussed while others feel that the label is going to be inaccurate, stigmatizing, and unhelpful.

There are a lot of different suggestions that are given for this name but they all work in order to try and make the sufferer not seem like they are such a harm to society or that they are going to cause more issues compared to other disorders. Coming up with the name that is going to work the best for describing the event is going to take some time. This is because the causes and reasons for having this disorder is going to be a bit different for each person who is involved. But the idea behind this is to help out those with the disorder so that they can get the help that they need without people having preconceived notions about their disorder ahead of time.

Chapter 8: Society and Culture: How they have portrayed this Disorder to the Mass Population

Most of the ideas that come with this disorder for the mass population come from the culture that is around it and the films and shows that have it. This is a big part of the way that people view this kind of disorder which might be some of the reason that it is so misunderstood. This section is going to spend a bit of time discussing some of the ways that borderline personality disorder has been portrayed in popular society to help determine why it may be looked down on with such stigmas as what are discussed in the previous chapter.

Television and Film

There are a lot of films and shows that you can find that are going to talk about this kind of disorder. In them they will either show someone who has been diagnosed with this type of disorder or they will show someone who has some of the traits of the disorder. Some of the shows and movies that show these kinds of traits include:

- Girl, Interrupted and Play Misty for Me—both of these movies are suggesting that there is a disorder about emotional instability. In the first one, there is a person who is showing aggressive behaviors to others rather than herself, which does not happen with BPD.

- The Sopranos—in this series, the therapist for the family suggests that the mother may be suffering from this disorder and even takes some time to quote the definition that is given to this disorder in the DSM. The character does seem to show a lot of the right traits which shows a shift in how this disorder is shown in many movies and shows.

- Will and Grace—while no one in this show has the disorder, the main character, Grace, tries to get her roommate, Will Truman, to forge a signature on a note that she has BPD as well as being at a higher risk for a psychotic break. While these two do not go together that much, the use of them together seems to show viewers that they are going to come together and that the disorder is going to show some psychotic break at some point.

- Star Wars—several psychiatrists have stated that the character of Anakin Skywalker is going to meet six out of the nigh criteria for diagnosing this disorder in a person. Some of the points to show for this include dissociative episodes, and uncertainty over who he was, and abandonment issues.
- The Cable Guy
- Fatal Attraction
- Notes on a Sandal
- A Thin Line Between Love and Hate

While there are a lot of examples of this kind of disorder to be found, it is often not done in a way that is showing the disorder in the right light. For the most part, when it is shown in shows and in the movies, the disorder has someone who is crazy, manipulative, liars, and who are going to have a break in any moment. It does not show the complexities that actually come with this disorder and often it makes people really misunderstand what is going on in this situation for the sufferer.

Literature

There is not that much in terms of literature that is about this kind of disorder outside of personal memoirs and nonfiction books about the disorder. Most of the time there is not much in terms of characters throughout history, though there might be a few. Some of the books that talk about this disorder include:

- Girl, Interrupted—not only is this a movie that shows a bit about the disorder, it is also a book that started it out first. This was written by Susanna Kaysen, an American author who was diagnosed with this disorder during the 1960s. This disorder was even less understood back then and often there was not much treatment options or it was not diagnosed right in the first place. This book describes what happens to the person who is diagnosed with the disorder and how they are treated and understood by others

- *Get Me Out of Here: My Recovery from Borderline Personality Disorder*—This is another memoir that was written by Rachel Reiland. It takes some time to talk about the time that she spent with treatment as well as recovery when she found out that she had borderline personality disorder.

- *Songs of Three Islands*—another memoir that was written by Millicent Monks, talks about how this personality disorder was impacting the Carnegie family when it started to show up. Instead of talking about her own issues with borderline personality disorder, she spends some time talking about a well-known family in American history and how they were affected by this disorder as well. While it may have been a great new look at the downfall of this family, many people have complained that it shed a really bad and biased light on the disorder and blamed it for a lot of things that just were not true. This makes a lot of people not like the book because of the inaccuracies as well as many people not really understand what is going on with this kind of disorder to those who have it.

- Komarr—this is one of the few fiction novels that talks about the disorder at all. This is a science fiction novel where the main character, according to the author, who has this personality disorder and this disorder is the thing that is driving a lot of what happens in the story. This is a unique way to look at the disorder and to begin to understand it a bit more.

Just like with the movies, most of the representations of this kind of disorder are done in the wrong way and can leave people feeling lost and confused as to what is really going on in the disorder. While some of the memoirs can help, the other options are not going to work as well and could leave the person with a lot to want when it comes to understanding this disorder. Many researchers believe that these portrayals, often the only interaction that people have with this disorder, can make it seem like it is something that it is not.

While these books and movies can give a little introduction to what is going on with this disorder it is important to realize that that they are not always the most accurate depictions of what is going on. It is better to take it and learn the information based off what you already know. The books and movies will also work in order to sensationalize the disorder, this one and many others, in order to make them sound better for the story so keep this in mind as well when you are watching and reading this information.

Conclusion

Dealing with the facts about borderline personality disorder is not something that anyone wants to deal with. It can be hard on everyone who is involved. The person who is going through this disorder is acting out and behaving in a way that they think they should because this is the only think that they know how to do. On the other hand, the behavior is not going to make any sense to the family and friends who are close to this person because they are the ones who are getting hurt in the process. Feelings can be wounded on either side, but after looking through this guidebook, it is easier to see why the person with this disorder is acting out in the way that they have been for so many years.

This is a complicated disorder and not one that should be taken lightly. The person who has been going through this disorder is going to need all of the help and support that they can get in order to get to a full recovery. It is not an easy process since many of the chemicals and thoughts that are in their own brain are the ones who are influencing the behavior that is there. But treatment is the only way to get them the help that they need to feel better and get back to their normal life with their friends and family.

The friends and family can work together with the person with the borderline personality disorder by offering to be supportive and be there when they are going through therapy. They can also work to get some of their own therapy to ensure that they are doing just fine in the process as well. This is not easy for either, but placing the blame on your loved one is just going to make the whole thing a lot worse to deal with. Being together is the best way for everyone to get through it.

Understanding what is going on with this disorder is often the first step. Most of the families who find out that a loved one has this personality disorder will often become more upset or mad at the person than they were before the diagnosis. This is often due to the fact that they do not understand the disorder and they assume that the person is lying to them, hiding something, or that nothing is actually wrong with them. Not only is the family guilty of this, but the person with the disorder may be feeling the same way which is why they may be so against getting the help they need.

This guidebook is meant to give much of the information that those with the disorder as well as their family members and friends are going to need in order to make it through this hard time. The person is often trying to get through something troubling that occurred in their childhood and this is not as easy as some may think. It takes a long time, perhaps years or more, to get it figured out, but with the right understanding and support, they are going to make it through just fine. In fact, the majority of those who get the treatment they need and stick with it are able to return to a normal life with their family and friends and they will not have a relapse ever after they are done.

Use this guidebook to get started on your understanding of this disorder. There is a lot to it and sometimes it is easy to get borderline personality disorder mixed up with one of the other disorders that are out there. This guidebook worked to try and get some of the misconceptions straightened out so that it is easier to understand what is going on and how the sufferer can be helped the most. If you or someone you know is going through this disorder, it is best to get them the help that they need right away. Using this guidebook is one of the best ways possible to help them out and get them back to the life that they deserve.

www.ingramcontent.com/pod-product-compliance
Lightning Source LLC
Chambersburg PA
CBHW070852290526
45795CB00001B/95